HIV Positive

HIV Positive
Perspectives on Counseling

Edited by

Margot Tallmer, PhD
Christopher Clason
Robert F. Lampke, MD
Dr. Austin H. Kutscher
Esther Braun, MSW, ACSW
Florence E. Selder, PhD, RN

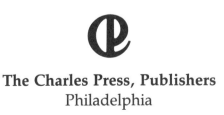

The Charles Press, Publishers
Philadelphia

The Charles Press, Publishers
Post Office Box 15715
Philadelphia, PA 19103

Library of Congress Cataloging-in-Publication Data

HIV positive: perspectives on counseling / edited by Margot Tallmer . . . [et al.].
     p.   cm.
  ISBN 0-914783-51-3 (pbk.)
  1. AIDS (Disease)—Patients—Counseling of.   1. Tallmer, Margot.   [DNLM: 1. Acquired Immunodeficiency Syndrome. 2. Counseling.   3. HIV Seropositivity.   WD 308 H6765]
RC607.A26H577   1990
362.1'969792—dc20
DNLM/DLC
for Library of Congress   90-15017
                                                                            CIP

Printed in the United States of America

ISBN 0-914783-51-3 (pbk.)

Editors

Margot Tallmer, PhD
Professor, Brookdale Center on Aging, Hunter College–City
University of New York, New York, New York

Christopher Clason
Executive Director, TPA Network, Inc., Chicago, Illinois

Robert F. Lampke, MD
Assistant Clinical Professor of Psychiatry, State University of New
York Health Sciences Center, Brooklyn, New York; Attending
Psychiatrist, Consultation Liaison Service, State University of New
York Hospital, Brooklyn, New York

Dr. Austin H. Kutscher
President, The Foundation of Thanatology, New York, New York;
Department of Psychiatry, College of Physicians and Surgeons,
Columbia University, New York, New York

Esther Braun, MSW, ACSW
Formerly, Medical Social Worker, Presbyterian Hospital, New York,
New York

Florence E. Selder, PhD, RN
Associate Professor of Nursing, University of Wisconsin School of
Nursing, Milwaukee, Wisconsin

Contributors

Janet D. Allan, RN, PhD
Assistant Professor in Nursing, University of Texas at Austin, Austin, Texas

Peter I. Bergé, PA-C, BS
Certified Physician Assistant, Division of Infectious Diseases, Beth Israel Medical Center, New York, New York

Cynthia Pike Blocksom, MEd, RD, LD
Training Coordinator, Cincinnati Health Department, Cincinnati, Ohio

Louise Boedeker, PhD
Associate Professor of Curriculum and Teaching, Hunter College–City University of New York; Co-founder, Center for Attitudinal Healing of New York City, New York, New York

Todd Butler (deceased)
Milwaukee, Wisconsin

Constance Captain, RN, PhD
Associate Chief of Nursing Service Research, Audie Murphy Veterans Memorial Hospital, San Antonio, Texas

Tony W. Cheung, MD, FACP
Physician-in-Charge, Division of Immunology and AIDS Program, Queens Hospital Center Affiliation of the Long Island Jewish Medical Center, Jamaica, New York

Seymour E. Coopersmith, EdD
President and Faculty-in-Training Analyst, National Association for Psychoanalysis, New York, New York

Ivan K. Goldberg, MD
Associate Attending Psychiatrist, Presbyterian Hospital; Associate in Clinical Psychiatry, Department of Psychiatry, College of Physicians and Surgeons, Columbia University, New York, New York

Judith Grad, JD
President, Metropolitan Institute for Training in Psychoanalytic Psychotherapy; formerly, Counsel to the New York City Board of Ethics, New York, New York

Beverly A. Hall, RN, PhD, FAAN
Denton and Louise Cooley Centennial Professor in Nursing, University of Texas at Austin, Austin, Texas

David Lester, PhD
Professor of Psychology, Richard Stockton State College, Pomona, New Jersey; formerly, Director of Research and Evaluation, Suicide Prevention Center of Buffalo, Buffalo, New York

Tom McGovern, EdD
Associate Professor of Psychiatry; Director, Bioethics-Humanities Program, Texas Tech Health Sciences Center, Lubbock, Texas

Mary B. McRae, EdD
Assistant Professor of Counseling, Department of Educational Foundations and Counseling Programs, Hunter College–City University of New York, New York, New York

"Michael"
Milwaukee, Wisconsin

Kathleen M. Nokes, PhD, RN
Assistant Professor of Nursing, Hunter College–Bellevue School of Nursing, New York, New York; Nurse Clinician, Bushwick Health Center and Woodhull Hospital and Mental Health Center, New York

Joyce S. Otten (deceased)
Freelance Writer, Battle Creek, Michigan

Rev. Jennifer Phillips, PhD
Chaplain, Brigham and Women's Hospital and Dana Farber Cancer Institute; former Chair, Ecumenical Task Force on AIDS, Boston, Massachusetts

Anthony Pilla, RN, BSN
Staff Nurse, Veterans Administration Hospital, New York, New York

Alan Rice, CSW
Adminstrative Supervisor, Department of Social Work, AIDS
Program, Beth Israel Medical Center, New York, New York

Tony Rizzolo
New York, New York

Fred Rosner, MD, FACP
Director, Department of Medicine, Queens Hospital Center Affilia-
tion of the Long Island Jewish Medical Center, Jamaica, New York;
Professor of Medicine, Health Sciences Center, State University of
New York at Stony Brook, Stony Brook, New York

Florence E. Selder, PhD, RN
Associate Professor of Nursing, University of Wisconsin School of
Nursing, Milwaukee, Wisconsin

Raphella Sohier, PhD, RN
Associate Professor of Nursing, Graduate Program in Nursing, University of Oklahoma, Norman, Oklahoma

Margot Tallmer, PhD
Professor, Brookdale Center on Aging, Hunter College–City University of New York, New York, New York

Eulon Ross Taylor, MD
Assistant Professor of Psychiatry; Co-Director, Bioethics-Humanities
Program, Texas Tech Health Sciences Center, Lubbock, Texas

Karyn Teufel
Milwaukee, Wisconsin

Contents

1

The AIDS Epidemic

Margot Tallmer, PhD

AIDS: DEFINITION

AIDS is a terminal, progressive infectious condition whose causative agent is called HIV, a slow-working human immunodeficiency retrovirus acquired through three major means of transmission: intrauterine exposure, before, during or right after childbirth; exchange of blood fluids or blood products, semen, or vaginal secretions; and by the use of contaminated needles or syringes. HIV in saliva is so minimal that infection by this route is virtually impossible. The virus, which by definition is symbiotic, that is, existing only within other living cells, compromises cellular immunity by killing white blood cells, and T-helper cells, thereby rendering the host organism prey to various opportunistic infections and Kaposi's sarcoma. These latter infections might be ordinarily warded off, withstood, or might not develop at all, they might also be long-time residents in the body which can now emerge when the immune effectiveness decreases. Opportunistic infections are generally of such severity that they cause death within three years after the diagnosis of AIDS is established. A diagnosis of AIDS is made after detecting HIV antibodies, and taking into account the clinical picture.

The Centers for Disease Control have established the following diagnostic criteria:

1. A positive blood test for serum antibodies to the virus that causes AIDS, or a positive cell culture for the virus.
2. A low number of T-helper white blood cells and a low ratio of T-helper white blood cells to T-suppressor white blood cells.
3. The presence of one or more opportunistic infections, indicative of immunodeficiency (Dalton 1987).

The two most common opportunistic infections are *Pneumocystis carinii* pneumonia, a protozoan infection of the lungs accounting for the largest percentage of AIDS deaths, and secondly, Kaposi's sarcoma, an extremely rare form of skin cancer diagnosed for the most part in gay or bisexual men with AIDS. Other infections are protozoal (pneumonia, encephalitis, enterocolitis), fungal (stomatitis, esophagitis, meningitis), bacterial (systemic infections) and viral (herpes simplex, herpes vulgaris, Epstein-Barr).

The cause of AIDS then is a virus, not misbehavior, but the initial stress on the risk to homosexuals and the connection to anal intercourse have offered reactionaries, like preacher Jerry Falwell, their own opportunistic infection—a chance to blame the victim and AIDS as appropriate divine punishment for offensive, unnatural sexual activities. Stigmatization of the victims extends to the media, nurses (Douglas et al. 1985), physicians (Douglas et al. 1985), nursing homes, employers, and gays themselves (Hays and Lyles 1986). The latter group, the gays, are accused of overstressing AIDS: "it is because identifying with sexually transmitted death plays to some dark belief that we deserve it" (*The Nation* 1989).

AFTER TESTING POSITIVE FOR THE HIV VIRUS

There are different possibilities after a person tests positive for the HIV virus. The blood test reveals antibodies to HIV usually about 2 to 3 months after infection. This is now a lifelong state in which the disease can be transmitted from one person to another. Casual contact (toilets, drinking glasses, kissing) does not provide a possible route, but only the three pathways mentioned earlier allow transmission. *There is no physical reason for refusing employment, health care, food service, or housing for those who are seropositive, have ARC, or have AIDS.*

The reasons for going on from an asymptomatic seropositive status to ARC (AIDS-related complex) are not well understood; only a certain percentage of ARC-infected persons develop AIDS; the timing between getting AIDS and death is also highly variable (Solomon and Temoshook 1987). Other viral infections, drug use, and nutrition are among potential variables that affect the course of illness (Kaplan et al. 1987). The Gay Men's Health Crisis estimates that 25 to 50% of confirmed seropositives will eventually develop AIDS within 5 to 10 years. A small number of seropositives have been free of illness for as long as 10 years.

The latest estimates of the Center for Disease Control are that only 1% of those seropositive will *not* develop AIDS (Lui, Darrow, and Rutherford 1988). This study, which was done in a San Francisco clinic for sexually transmitted diseases, compared this sample with those who have become seropositive through blood transfusions. Batchelor

(1988) feels the results of Lui's study are grossly exaggerated, for the gay group had very high sexual activity, had come to a clinic for sexually transmitted diseases rather than to their regular physicians, and had been attracted to the study because of a history of such diseases. Furthermore, they lived in a city with a high incidence of AIDS.

The Gay Men's Health Crisis notes that there is too little survey data of the general population and that wide variations within communities in the prevalence of the disease and of those testing positive must be studied in the context of location, age of the sampled , and the frequency of high-risk behavior. The HIV virus was introduced in different places at different times. Even now the virus is still so young that extrapolations remain difficult. One may be seropositive without any symptoms, but unfortunately, the longer the time lapse since testing HIV positive, the greater the chance of being infected with AIDS.

Some people do develop serious conditions but not AIDS, for example, ARC, sometimes termed HIV-related illness or HIV-associated disease, wherein several of the symptoms associated with AIDS are present but not the opportunistic infections or Kaposi's sarcoma.

The Centers for Disease Control have established the following criteria for ARC:

1. The presence of two of these signs for a period of at least 3 months:
   unexplained weight loss, fever, swollen lymph nodes, severe diarrhea, drenching night sweats, yeast infections, severe fatique.
2. Two laboratory findings:
   (a) low number of T-helper white blood cells which activate the specific disease-fighting cells and instruct the creation of antibodies that rid the body of microscopic invaders;
   (b) low ratio of T-helper to T-suppressor cells (which can tell the immune system when the threat is over).
3. One of the following:
   low red or low white blood cell count, low platelet count, elevated levels of serum globulins (infection-fighting proteins).

Supposedly ARC affects 10 to 100 (estimates vary) times as many persons as does AIDS; a proportion, of unknown size, of persons with ARC will progress to AIDS.

Although there is uncertainty about the physiological routes after seropositive testing, the psychological effects seem less hypothetical.

The initial stresses of deciding to have the test performed, awaiting results, and the return for a second validation, may be overlooked if the results are favorable. There are no hard data yet as to whether risk-taking sexual behavior decreases in this event. But if results are unfavorable, one is immediately faced with an uncertain future that will include the need for continual periodic monitoring and treatment, possible economic upheaval, physical crises, identification with a discredited high-risk group, public admission of a sexual orientation that may have been a past secret, and the frightening, sobering recognition of mortality. We know from work on crisis intervention that faced with such an overwhelming experience, one must and will solve the crisis. The issue is how beneficial the solution is. Does one hopefully grow and profitably gain from the experience? Or is one faced with a lack of any resource in the psychological armamentarium that will assist in coping?

We also know from crisis work that stress, with affective changes, has immunological consequences. Bereavement, loneliness, and loss have been shown to decrease immunological strength (Bartrop et al. 1977, Schliefer et al. 1983, Irwin et al. 1987). These psychosocial variables are additional possibilities for affecting HIV infection and disease progression (Kiecolt-Glaser and Glaser 1988). Research on aging has demonstrated that ill health is the greatest predictor of disengagement in the elderly (Tallmer and Kutner 1980) and that there is a higher degree of mortality in the isolated (Cohen and Syme 1985). Feelings of loss, separation and isolation are common incomitants of people designated as ill; women separated less than a year had poorer immunological functioning than did married counterparts (Kiecolt-Glaser et al. 1987) and this is also true for men (Kiecolt-Glaser et al. 1988); in fact, marital disruption is the single most important factor in predicting physical and emotional illnesses (Somers 1979).

We acknowledge the direct and indirect effects of behavior on the immune system. Cautious psychosocial interventions should expectedly impact on the HIV virus and the patient's waning immunological strength. Additionally, the fear, burnout, exhaustion, anticipatory grief, and anger of the caregivers are readily observable and must impinge on the psychological interface between the ill and the well. Such interrelationships are also open to positive psychotherapeutic strategies that may ameliorate the tensions between the two.

Continuous, chronic stress, often inducing anxiety, anger and depression, does not appear to favor immunological immunity and over extended periods of time apparently causes a decrease in immunologic regulation (Kiecolt-Glaser et al. 1987). Intervention is necessary because we are unable to stop the downward trend.

HISTORY OF AIDS

A Danish woman surgeon, stationed in Zaire, had actually demonstrated symptoms of AIDS as early as 1976, and for a time Africa became linked with the origin of the disease. It was not until 5 years later, 1981, that the first case of AIDS in the United States was formally reported to the Centers for Disease Control. But earlier, alert physicians had begun recognizing a new syndrome in a small number of relatively young, previously healthy male patients—a prolonged, debilitating illness that began with vague, ill-defined symptoms that led to persistent mysterious deterioration and eventually progressed to death. On examination, the state of their nearly powerless immune systems closely resembled systems affected by carcinomas or drugs used to suppress the rejection of organ transplants.

Going even further back in time, troubling questions had surfaced concerning health problems in male homosexuals. A disproportionately high number of them suffered bouts of amoebic dysentery, amebiasis, giardiasis, venereal diseases, and hepatitis B. In 1978, for example, a large sample of gay men were tested in San Francisco; 1% had antibodies to HIV, by 1980 the number had increased to 25%, and by 1984 had reached 65%.

Because of the high incidence of Kaposi's sarcoma (originally thought to affect only older Jewish and Italian men and rarely seen in the U.S.), the disease was labeled KS/01, then GRID (an acronym for Gay-Related Immune Deficiency). The obvious distaste for such a pejorative label led to the final choice of a more comfortable term, an acronym less shrouded in sexuality, since the use of the word "acquired" implies that its cause is external and as yet unknown (Shilts 1987, p. 171). (One might argue that "acquired" could be viewed as caused by misbehavior, "acquired" through undesirable acts.)

Belatedly, the search for a virus began—a virus that produces little disease in itself but weakens resistance to other ailments. Once the virus was uncovered, viral antigens could be produced on a large scale, and a test might be found to detect the presence of virus-induced antibodies in the system. HIV is actually a retrovirus. Known to us for only about 9 years, retroviruses are composed only of genetic material, that is, RNA (ribonucleic acid) and carry enzymes that permit DNA to be bypassed, for they can copy RNA with DNA. Robert Gallo showed that there was some connection between this retrovirus and the T cells. T cells are involved in cellular inactivity and leukemia. The retrovirus becomes part of and hidden in the DNA of the T-4 cells.

Precious time elapsed while public attention and government funds were directed elsewhere. Even when the search for the virus was in full swing, the investigation was marked by national and international competition, political overtones, and stigmatization of the victims. Once linked to homosexuality, the search was hampered by a pervasive ignorance of male homosexual practices (Batchelor 1988). If doctors have a hard time dealing with death (and they often do), this type of fatal illness engendered even more anxiety and prejudice. To know a disease is transmitted through sexual behavior is to be faced with a lack of data—nothing on a large-scale basis had been done since Kinsey.

We know from Watson and Crick's revelations on the backstage life of the discovery of DNA that science is scarcely free of the political tensions that seem to affect us all, but unlike the remarkable DNA work which they did and which had such far-reaching implications, the delayed programs due to prejudice, disdain, and lack of interest permitted the epidemic to spread. Many unnecessary deaths have occurred. Early on, the political air was fatally polluted by public reactions to buzz words such as anal intercourse, homosexuality, sleazy bath house practices, and promiscuity. And, of course, AIDS is associated very clearly straight on, with death, epidemics, and unknown incubation periods (Herek and Glunt 1988).

Some of the major events in the uncovering of the virus include the following:

1. In 1980, Dr. Robert Gallo, an American, reported a confirmed isolation of a retrovirus, HILV-III, from humus which conformed to lymphocytes of the T type which controls cell-mediated immunity.

2. In 1983, at the Pasteur Institute in Paris, Dr. Luc Montagnier headed a team that proclaimed the discovery of the AIDS virus, and called it LAV, or lymphadenopathy-associated virus. At that time, a lawsuit was filed for recognition of this discovery, disputing the National Cancer Institute's and Dr. Gallo's claim to being first.

3. Also in 1983, J.C. Chermann and Luc Montagnier studied the cells of gay men with lymphadenopathy syndrome, believing that AIDS was a final stage of LAS.

4. Dr. Jonas Salk undertook a Kissinger-like shuttle diplomacy between France and America and a compromise was reached. The Committee for Taxonomy of Viruses, an international group, finally declared that AIDS was not a leukemia virus (AIDS victims do not customarily get leukemia, but have the same subset of T cells that give rise to leukemia of HTLV-1) and the committee finally settled upon HIV; Presidents Reagan and Chirac of France co-signed the compromise citing Gallo and Montagnier as co-discoverers.

5. Finally, the American National Cancer Institute and National Red Cross together worked on a test for HIV antibodies—a test which

immediately evoked concerns regarding civil liberties, protecting public health, confidentiality, accuracy, and medical ethics. In passing, it should be noted that the blood banks, deploring the expense, resisted testing even when the virus was demonstrably able to be transmitted through the exchange of blood products containing Factor VIII, a substance that permits clotting, and whole blood. Factor VIII was a product of thousands of donors, filtered, concentrated and then injected into the hemophiliac recipient. By 1982, it became apparent that Factor VIII, during the preparation procedure, could not filter out Pneumocystis. Although hemophiliacs accounted for only a small proportion of (2%) of total AIDS victims, action was clearly mandated to avoid economic disaster, as if moral concerns were not sufficient. Blood banks are exactly that—banks—large, private, competitive businesses with many financial resources that might fuel the basis for lawsuits. Since the people infected with the transfusion-related HIV virus were objects of public sympathy, in no way censured for their sexual misbehavior, and were not hidden from society, they would be more likely to be successful in seeking legal compensation (although all AIDS sufferers are certainly victims, the public could see them as "true victims"!). Blood banks could be charged with "failure to exercise reasonable care in administering or producing blood" (Dalton 1987, p. 168). Blood banks resolutely resisted testing, although they ultimately agreed that persons demonstrating direct manifestation of AIDS could not donate. The banks refused to reveal the names of donors, even when transmission by blood donation was evidenced and would not permit any contact with the donors, whom the banks would, by telephone, question about possible risks. Homosexuals were actually a substantial part of the donor pool, and gay groups rallied in the condemnation of any screening. Screening implied possible discrimination, posed a threat to confidentiality and health insurance, was based on sexual orientation, and might ultimately lead to segregation, even quarantine (Shilts 1987). At this point in time, 1983, no test for HIV antibodies existed but testing for hepatitis core antibodies would help screen out high-risk donors.

By 1984, there were 74 cases of AIDS that were related to blood transfusions and of these, 73 were hemophiliacs. Irwin Memorial Bank, in San Francisco, high in the distribution of AIDS-infected blood, announced that, alone in the blood industry, they would begin testing their blood for antibodies to AIDS, using a test licensed by the Abbott Laboratories. Testing issues were clouded by concerns for civil liberties, financial pressures, the use of blood banks as a diagnostic tool, and the medical value of the test. Fears about the test were prevalent in the gay community and unfortunately, not completely unfounded. Health insurers, for example, have certainly been interested in test results. A *New York Times* headline (August 7, 1989) proclaimed that "Insurance Limits Growing to Curb AIDS Coverage" and cited the hardships persons with AIDS face in obtaining and retaining health, disability, and life insurance. But mass gay opposititon was decreased when the government agreed both to pay for alternative test sites, and not to use the test as a screening of groups at risk.

The tests—all use the ELISA techniques (enzyme-linked immunosorbent assay)—are 95% (93–99%) sensitive; sensitivity is the ability of the test to identify people with the condition. Nineteen out of twenty persons infected with the virus would be detected. The test is 99% specific; specificity is the ability of the test to identify people who do not have the condition. Ninety-nine times out of a hundred, the test would not produce a false antibody-positive result. Clearly, a false positive would not be a major problem in screening blood; one would just not use that sample.

But there is actually little research on the sensitivity and specificity of the various ELISA tests. The test is very accurate in screening blood donations because it is a self-selected sample—high-risk donors have been eliminated. Similarly, high-risk persons taking the test can also be confident since the test is most accurate when the prevalence of seropositivity is high. As an overall large-scale screening device, although inexpensive, ELISA is not useful because of the low prevalence. Only a small percentage of people have HIV virus. Predictive value is then only 50%, with a large number of false positives. Therefore, one must repeat a positive result, usually using the Western blot, a more difficult, costly and time consuming method. A false positive may be due to contamination, technical error, or confounding medical conditions. A false positive can manifestly cause immeasurable anguish and discrimination. We repeat, a test can only support a diagnosis; it cannot identify AIDS or ARC, nor does it mean one will eventually develop those illnesses. Finally, the test cannot identify antibodies until 6 weeks after infection, and possibly not before a year. HIV-positive status can eventuate in a variety of conditions, causing damage not only to the immune syustem but also the brain and central nervous system (Hoffman et al. 1984) and thus lead to organically based depression. The issue is that of what one does with the results. Does the testing affect behavioral change? (Coates et al. 1988). Many do not want to know the results, (Lyter et al. 1987) anticipating depression and anxiety. Others feel the knowledge can help them cope better and reduce their high-risk behavior. There is no cure and no vaccine and no one has recovered from AIDS. Our hopes are that voluntary healthy behavioral changes will prevent further spread of this disease.

DEMOGRAPHICS

Specific demographics and future projections about the epidemic of AIDS vary drastically, muddying the possibilities for future planning. Some health officials are astoundingly sanguine while others paint a bleak, frightening canvas. A headline in a *New York Times* article reads "A Tenfold Rise in AIDS is Seen." "The World Health Organization predicted that the total number of AIDS cases would increase from 400,000 today to 5,000,000 by the year 2000, and that those infected with HIV would increase three times from the present count of between 5 and 10 million."

There are actually no hard data on the prevalence of AIDS today, but the Centers for Disease Control put the figure at somewhere between 1 and 1.5 million American men, women and children who are infected with the HIV virus; perhaps, internationally, the figure would reach 5 million (World Health Organization). Most of the AIDS cases, presumably about one quarter of the total (about 400,000) live in New York City. New cases of AIDS appear at the rate of 100 per day throughout the country. Early on in the epidemic, 75% of those infected were white gay or bisexual men—leading to the pejorative terms "gay plague" and "WOG" [Wrath of God]; gays are still the largest high-risk group. Sexual patterns among gays are changing. For example, in San Francisco, gay men who were exposed to a prevention model to change high-risk behavior have refrained from AIDS-related sexual activity to a greater degree than anywhere else in our country (Coates et al. 1988). There has been a decrease in new cases reported there for 2 years now. Thus, statistics on the gay groups must be watched carefully to see which models should be developed for risk reduction. The percentage of homosexual-related AIDS has dropped from 77% to 70% of all cases and continues to decline. Shilts (1987) feels that the press did not even cover AIDS with any degree of appropriateness as long as it was considered a gay disease. Other high-risk groups emerged later among the heterosexual, intravenous drug user, and female populations. The spread of AIDS among heterosexuals appears to be slower than among gays. Heterosexual partners of AIDS-infected persons make up 4% of all cases (Brooks Gunn, Boyer, and Hein 1988). "HIV is neither very infectious, nor very contagious; that is, it is difficult to transmit from one person to another and it does not easily survive in the body once it is transmitted" (Batchelor 1988).

Notwithstanding this disclaimer, and the fact that preventive methods do not involve a great deal of expense (condoms, bleach), AIDS has spread in epidemic proportions throughout the world, through heterosexual sex, IV drug use, and medical procedures; for example, in many countries, needles for injections are regularly reused because of the expense and limited supply. The geographical data are quite varied; in Spain and Italy, the largest number of AIDS cases is reported in IV drug users, while in many parts of the world, such as Central Africa, AIDS is now primarily a heterosexual disease transmitted male-to-female, or female-to-male, and appears with equal frequency in both sexes.

AIDS ranks eighth in the years of potential life lost (CDC 1986) and is the only cause of death that continues to rise each year.

SPECIAL GROUPS

Drug Users

AIDS among drug users in the U.S. is increasing, accounting for 21% of the total, with highest percentages in the northeastern region of the country. The greatest threat to contracting AIDS is for people who are, in any way, part of the drug scene. After gays, they make up the second largest group with AIDS in our country, and transmit the virus to women and children (Des Jarlais and Friedman 1988). Certainly, some women are drug users themselves (albeit a small percentage) and some have had contact with infected men. The woman IV drug user is probably in the social milieu wherein sexual intercourse would take place with another drug user. If new sterilized needles are unavailable either because of the legal system or financial resources, they are likely to share equipment or go to "shooting galleries" that provide drug paraphernalia.

It is a given that drug users less frequently have health insurance, with consequent loss of access to the medical system, and are often victims of racial discrimination. There are about 1/2 million addicts in our country, with about 50% living in New York City. Any demographic data about drug users will inherently be compounded by the variables of race and gender, which are in turn affected by socioeconomic status, education, attitudes about the self, and discrimination. Finally, 7% of AIDS patients fit two categories, being gay and drug users, blacks and Hispanics.

We do know that blacks and Hispanics are disproportionately represented in all categories except hemophiliacs, that they contract AIDS at least three times as frequently as whites for homosexual and bisexual men, and twenty times more frequently than whites for heterosexual black and Hispanic men. One half of the infected minority members are heterosexual drug users. Ethnic minorities comprise 40% of the total AIDS cases: 24% are black and 14% Hispanic.

The variables that must be considered in minority AIDS patients are difficult to exclude from any research design. There are the obvious ones that we have cited for drug users. There are less easily measured attitudes that affect the spread of the disease, such as sexual preferences among minority members, the influence of macho thinking, and the integration of minority members into a social system that provides intervention, information and support. Minority men, for example, may opt for both homosexual and heterosexual activities (the number of bisexual cases reported by the Centers for Disease Control was divided into 31% black, 20% Hispanic and 13% white); they may use prostitution more frequently (Peterson and Marin 1988)—minority prostitutes test positive for HIV more often than their white counterparts (Carrier 1985)—and they may be victimized by homophobia more often than whites.

In terms of drug use, blacks and Hispanics more frequently share drug equipment than white drug users (Des Jarlais et al. 1988).

Hemophiliacs

Blood screening has been in place since 1986, so that hemophiliacs should no longer be at risk. By 1988, 1 in 26 hemophiliacs has contracted AIDS; there are 20,000 hemophilacs through the U.S.(Mason, Olsen and Parish 1988, p. 971). Hemophiliacs are randomly distributed; there is no special ethnic group, geographical location, or socioeconomic factor typical of this category, making them an excellent sample for research purposes.

Children and Adolescents

As of May 1988, 900 children, less than 13 years old, have AIDS. Of these, 77% acquired it through perinatal transmission; the rest through blood products. The vast majority of pediatric cases (75%) are from New York, northern New Jersey and southern Florida (Brooks-Gunn, Bryer, and Hein 1988). Most children (80%) with AIDS are less than 5 years old; one-half are black, one-fifth white, and one-fifth Hispanic. In New York City one out of 61 babies test positive: 50% have HIV and 50% have picked up maternal antibodies. It is difficult to distinguish between the two possibilities.

In adolescents as compared to adults, there is a greater proportion of infected women, minority members, and heterosexuals. The numbers are low but rising. Perhaps this may be expected with this age-group, for risk-taking seems to be an integral part of puberty. Additionally, many young people are unable to think ahead or resist impulses.

Women

In 1988, there were 66,464 people with AIDS; 5,757 of these were women. Mays and Cochran (1988) estimate that there are 50,000 seropositive women in New York City. Fifty percent of those are drug users; 20% have sexual partners who are drug users. About 40,000 of the women are black or Hispanic. Between the ages of 25 and 29, AIDS is the leading cause of death in women (Kristal 1986).

These statistics are tragic and surprising, for AIDS is commonly thought of as a gay men's disease, and women have received attention chiefly as possible infectors, i.e., nursing mothers, prostitutes (Wolfsley 1987).

The proportion of female seropositives to the total pool has been increasing more rapidly than that of any other high-risk group. Within this subset, black and Hispanic women are at greatest risk.

Eighty percent of pediatric AIDS cases can be traced to the presence of the virus in the mother. Interestingly enough, many women, even when seropositive, do not choose to abort the baby. Asymptomatic HIV does not preclude conception, so that many mothers are unaware that they are positive for HIV when they conceive. Pregnancy accelerates the progress of the illness.

It is true that vaginal transmission has occurred from woman to man, and there is a reported case of a woman transmitting the disease to another woman. Generally, in sexual transmission, women receive the virus from a partner.

When infected, women become sicker and die of AIDS more quickly than men. The illness is not the same for both; for example, women rarely contract Kaposi's sarcoma.

Clearly, in cases of rape and incest where there may be cuts, bleeding, and bruises, the chances of contracting any infection are great.

REFERENCES

AIDS: A Social Work Response. 1987. Proposed Revised Social Policy Statement for the 1987 Delegate Assembly of the National Association of Social Workers.

Bakeman, R., E. McCray, J.R. Lumb, R.E. Jackson and P.N. Whitney. 1987. The incidence of AIDS among Black and Hispanics. *J.A.M.A.* 79:921–928.

Bartrolp, R.W., E. Luckhurst, L. Lazarus, L.G. Kiloh and R. Penny. 1977. Depressed lymphocyte function after bereavement. *Lancet* 1:834–836.

Batchelor, W.F. 1988. AIDS 1988: The science and the limits of science. *Am. Psycologist* 43,11, (November): 853–858.

Brooks-Gunn, J., C.B. Boyer and K. Hein. Preventing HIV infection and AIDS in children and adolescents. *Am. Psychologist* 43, 11:958–964.

Carnier, J.M. 1987. Mexican male bisexuality. In F. Klein and T.J. Wolf, eds., *Bisexualities; Theory and Research.* New York: Haworth Press.

Coates, T.J., R.D. Stall, and C.C. Hoff. Changes in sexual behavior of gay and bisexual men since the beginning of the AIDS epidemic. Washington, DC: U.S. Congress, Office of Technology Assessment.

Cohen, S. and S.L. Syme, eds., 1985. *Social Support and Health.* New York: Academic Press.

Dalton, H.L., S. Burris and the Yale AIDS Law Project. 1987. New Haven and London.

Des Jarlais, D.C., and S. Friedman. 1987. Target groups for preventing AIDS among intravenous drug users. *J. Applied Soc. Psychol.* 17:251–268.

Douglas, C.J., C.M. Kalman and T. P. Kalman. 1985. Homophobia among physicians and nurses: An empirical study. *Hospital Community Psychiatry* 36, 12 (December): 1309–1311.

Guinan, M.E. and A. Hardy. 1987. Epidemiology of AIDS in women in the United States. *J.A.M.A.* 257, 15:2039–2042.

Hays, L.R. and M.R. Lyles. 1986. Psychological themes in patients with AIDS. *Am. J. Psychiatry* 143, 4:551–553.

Herek, G.M. and E. Glunt. 1988. An epidemic of stigma. *Am. Psychologist* 43, 11:886–891.

Hoffman, R. 1984. Neuropsychiatric complications of AIDS. *Psychosomatics* 25, 5:393–400.

Irwin, M., M. Daniels, T.L. Smith, E. Bloom and H. Werner. 1987. Impaired natural killer cell activity during bereavement. *Brain, Behavior Immunity* 1:98–104.

Kaplan, H.B., R.J. Johnson, C.A. Bailey, and W. Simon. 1987. The sociological study of AIDS: A critical review of the literature and suggested research agenda. *J. Health Social Behav.* 28:140–157.

Kermani, B.J., J.C. Borod, P.H. Brown, and G. Tunnell. 1985. New psychopathologic findings in AIDS: Case report. *J. Clin. Psychiatry* 46, 6:240–241.

Kiecolt-Glaser, J.K., R. Glaser, C. Dyer, E. Shuttleworth, P. Ogrocki, and C.E. Spercher. 1987. Chronic stress and immunity in family caregivers of Alzheimer's disease victims. *Psychosomatic Med.* 49:523–535.

———. 1988. Psychological influences on immunity; Implications for AIDS. *Am. Psychologist* 43,11:892–898.

Kristal, A. 1986. The impact of the acquired immunodeficiency syndrome on patterns of premature death in New York City. *J.A.M.A.* 255:2306–2310.

Lui, K., W. Darrow, and G.W. Rutherford. 1988. A model-based estimate of the mean incubation period for AIDS in homosexual men. *Science* 240:1333–1335.

Lyter, D.W., R.O. Valdiserri, L.A. Kingsley, W.P. Ameros, and C.R. Rinaldo. 1987. The HIV antibody test: Why gay and bisexual men want or do not want their results. *Public Health Reports* 102:468–474.

Mason, P.J., R.A. Olson, and K.L. Parish. 1988. AIDS, hemophilia, and preventive efforts within a comprehensive care program. *Am. Psychologist* 43, 11:971–976.

Mass, L. 1987. *Medical Answers About AIDS.* New York: Gay Men's Health Crisis.

Mays, V.M. and S.D. Cochran. 1988. Issues in the perception of AIDS risk and risk reduction activities by black and Hispanic/Latina women. *Am. Psychologist* 43, 11:949–957.

McArthur, J.C. 1987. Neurologic manifestations of AIDS. *Medicine* 66:407–437.

Medical Answers About AIDS. 1988. L. Mass ed. New York: Gay Men's Health Crisis.

Morin, S.F. 1988. AIDS: The challenge of psychology. *Am. Psychologist* 43, 11:838–842.

Nation, AIDS as apocalypse, February 13, 1989.

New York City Chapter, National Association of Social Workers. Position Paper on Social Work Practice for People with AIDS, ARC, and HIV Infection, October 16, 1986.

New York Times, Friday, May 19, 1989.

Nurnberg. H.G., J. Prudic, M. Fiori, and E.P. Freedman. 1984. Psychopathology Complicating AIDS. *Am. J. Psychiatry* 141, 1:95–96.

Peterson, J.L. & G. Marin. 1988. Issues in the prevention of AIDS among Black and Hispanic men. *Am. Psychologist* 43, 11:871-876.

Scully, R.E., E.J. Mark, and B.U. McNeely. 1986. Case records of the Mass. General Hospital: Case 2. *N. Engl. J. Med.* 314:167–174.

Shilts, R. 1987. *And the Band Played On.* New York: Penguin Books.

Snider, W.D., D.M. Simpson, S. Nielsen, J.W.M. Gold, C.E. Metroka, and J.E. Posner. 1983. Neurological complications of acquired immunodeficiency syndrome: Analysis of 50 patients. *Ann. Neurol.* 14:403–418.

Solomon, G.F. and L. Temoshook. 1987. A psychoneuroimmunologic perspective on AIDS research: Questions, preliminary findings and suggestions. *J. Applied Soc. Psychol.* 17:286–308.

Somers, A.R. 1979. Marital status, health and use of health services. *J.A.M.A.* 241:1818–1822.

Tallmer, M. and B. Kutner. 1980. Disengagement and the stresses of aging in thanatologic aspects of aging. New York, unpublished.

Wofsy, C.B. 1987. Human immunodeficiency virus infection in women. *J.A.M.A.* 257:2074–2076.

2

The Short-Term Psychosocial Implications of HIV Antibody Test Results

Peter I. Bergé, PA-C, BS

The decision to be tested for antibodies to Human Immunodeficiency Virus (HIV), the agent associated with AIDS, can entail an emotional experience ranging from mild curiosity to extreme distress. Being tested can be an event as casual as donating blood, or it may involve weeks or months of internal struggle, discussions with friends, partners, and family; and consultation with therapists, physicians, and even attorneys. Testing is performed in a variety of settings, such as medical offices, hospitals, military infirmaries (screening of recruits), health department testing sites, blood collection and processing centers, and in clinics specializing in sexually transmitted diseases, family planning, and intravenous substance abuse. The process traditionally consists of pre-test counseling, blood-drawing, a wait of several days to a few weeks for the result to come back, revelation of the result to the person being tested, and post-test counseling. This model does not pertain to the testing of donated blood since the tests are performed as part of the mass-screening of blood for safety purposes, and not as a service or part of medical evaluation.

In most states, highly confidential or anonymous testing is offered in "alternate test sites" (ATS) run or sponsored by health departments, and the pre- and post-test counseling may be carried out by specially trained lay personnel, nurses, or other public health staff. Testing and counseling are also available in some volunteer-staffed or other community-based, nonprofit service organizations serving populations in which there is a high rate of HIV infection. AIDS service organizations and public health departments have developed manuals and formal training programs for HIV-testing counselors in these settings, and some institutions conduct regular case reviews to enhance counseling skills, provide support, and share techniques for managing difficult situations.

In addition to the testing that is widely available through ATS centers, a substantial number of tests are ordered by independent medical care providers such as physicians, physician assistants, and nurse practitioners in other settings. In general, the training on HIV antibody test counseling that is most accessible to these medical providers is in the form of lectures and workshops as part of continuing education programs, and is not as structured nor as comprehensive as the courses given to the counselors mentioned previously. Additionally, some medical personnel who are highly trained in the biological aspects of HIV infection do not feel that they need additional education on the psychosocial dimensions of HIV counseling. The perspective of the counseling is likely to differ as well; lay counselors and mental health professionals are inclined to focus on emotional and social issues and to explicitly refrain from giving "medical advice." Medical clinicians, however, are accustomed to providing medical advice and concrete interventions; this is often the expectation when they are consulted by patients, and the contrast gives an entirely different quality to the counseling interaction.

People being tested for HIV antibodies may be divided into four categories: (1) those who wish to be tested because of a concern, realistic or not, about activities or events that might have resulted in infection (e.g., sexual contact, needle sharing, or exposure to someone else's blood in an open wound); (2) patients with symptoms that might be attributed to HIV infection, and in whom a positive test result might result in a diagnosis of symptomatic HIV disease (such as AIDS or AIDS-Related Complex [ARC]); (3) those who are required to submit to testing, such as military recruits, Peace Corps volunteers, immigrants, and (in some states) applicants for some types of insurance; and (4) those who are tested in connection with the donation of blood or blood products, many of whom give only a passing thought to the issue of testing. While the boundaries between these categories are in reality blurred, they are nonetheless useful when considering the varied responses to a positive test result.

The notification of HIV antibody-positive blood donors is a topic deserving of much more attention than can be given here. Nonetheless, it is important to state that the practice of donating blood in order to be tested is one which should be strongly discouraged, and this has been the position of the blood banking industry for several years (American Blood Commission Task Force on AIDS 1985). From the psychological perspective, there are two reasons for this: first, effective pre-test counseling cannot be performed in the "beltline" setting of a blood drive; second, the time until notification of a positive result may not be readily established, and those with negative results are not notified at all. Therefore, the notification of a positive test result may occur without any significant preparation and may challenge the resources of even the most skillful post-test counselors.

THE TEST

In simple terms, the HIV antibody test indicates whether or not there is laboratory evidence of infection with HIV. As defined here, a positive test is one in which a very sensitive screening test (called an ELISA, or EIA) is positive (reactive) two or more times, and in which that result was confirmed by a more specific test such as the Western blot. When these tests are performed by laboratories with large-volume experience and strict quality control, the results are extremely accurate and almost certainly indicate that HIV antibody is present (Centers for Disease Control 1988). Since it is current scientific opinion that this virus does not leave the body once infection occurs, the presence of HIV antibodies in the serum (HIV antibody seropositivity) must be taken as evidence that the virus is present as well (Centers for Disease Control 1987). A positive HIV antibody test, by itself, cannot give any indication of when the infection occurred, how much virus may be present, or the state of health of the patient; in the absence of other information the test cannot diagnose clinical AIDS, and should *never* be referred to as "the AIDS test."

A negative test means that HIV antibody could not be detected in the blood at the time of the test. Most often, this indicates that the person has not been infected with HIV. Alternately, it could mean that the test was done soon after infection occurred (a few weeks to 6 months) and that there has not been enough time for the production of detectable levels of antibody (Francis and Chin 1987). There have also been extremely rare instances in which people have failed to develop antibody for long periods of time after infection, or lost antibody for unexplained reasons (Barnes 1988, Wilber 1988); advanced AIDS can also account for loss of antibody as the immune system becomes ultimately depleted. An indeterminate, or inconclusive, test result occurs when the screen test (ELISA) is reactive and the confirmatory test (Western blot) shows a partial reaction which can not be interpreted as either positive or negative.

THE POSITIVE TEST RESULT

Initial Reactions

The patient's early reactions are often influenced by his or her expectations of the results, and by the context in which the test was performed. For example, the long-time sexual partner of someone who has recently died of AIDS may be unsurprised and accept the information with equanimity, while someone taking the test for a Peace Corps or insurance application who is not aware of any risk will be completely unprepared for the result. However, the medical provider cannot depend on membership in "high-risk groups" to predict the reaction to a positive test result. A gay man who has had few partners, practiced some degree of "safer sex," and lived in an area where there have been few reported cases of AIDS might be considered to be at low risk; he may be understandably shocked by a positive result. In other cases, denial is a potent influence on the expectation of a negative result: the woman whose partner had used intravenous (IV) drugs several years in the past may not wish to consider herself to be at risk; the IV drug user (IVDU) who only shares needles with close friends often does not see this as a dangerous activity. The man who identifies himself as heterosexual, but who has numerous risky sexual contacts with other men, is likely to feel that he is "safe" because he is "not gay." Many of those who have knowingly engaged in multiple high-risk behaviors may choose to interpret their continuing good health, and that of their partners, as an indication that they remain uninfected. Even if symptoms should be present (unexplained weight loss, fatigue, prolonged soaking night sweats, multiple enlarged lymph nodes, for instance) they, too, can be explained away in the denial process. In some of these situations the pretext for the testing may seem totally unrelated to the known risk or the symptoms, and when the patient expresses a strong reaction to the positive result, it reflects validation of the repressed fears that led to the testing.

Aside from the issue of surprise, a wide range of early reactions can be expected. When there is anger, it is often directed toward a partner, especially when the patient went for testing after finding out about the partner's history of high-risk activities. Guilt is very common, and is most pronounced when the patients have conflicts about whatever activities might have placed them at risk for infection. Sadness, fear, and despair are frequently manifested when patients equate the positive test with having AIDS, and AIDS with death. It often seems that the patient feels as if he or she has been awaiting a death decree, and begins to listen to the pronouncement of the sentence as soon as the result is given; it is not unusual for several minutes to pass (or even longer) before the patient is prepared to hear the clinician's words over the internal "tape" being played.

When depression seems to be an early reaction during the notification session, it is possible that the individual is already depressed for reasons unrelated to the test result. Concerns about suicidal risk, which must always be considered when giving a positive result, are even more pertinent in these cases. In other situations the news may be received impassively. A stoic reception of the positive test result, although it may be welcomed by the anxious clinician, should justly provoke uneasiness since it is most likely masking or postponing a much stronger reaction and making it harder to formulate helpful interventions. Denial, when it persists to this point, usually results in the validity of the test result being questioned, and repeat testing requested or sought in a different setting.

Finally, there are patients who express a sense of relief when learning that they are HIV seropositive. Many of these have long suspected that they had been infected with HIV, some have experienced symptoms, and most have suffered from the uncertainty of not definitively knowing where they stood. This is most likely to occur in people who are familiar with many support services for seropositives, and who then feel free to move on, avail themselves of those supports, and accept the new "identity" of being a seropositive, with its attendant sense of community.

RAMIFICATIONS

Loss

After the initial reactions, many patients will begin to grieve. This early process of grieving represents the many losses which the positive test result implies to them. It can be profoundly affecting to observe patients as they discover the many parts of their lives which are touched by this one event.

The most basic loss is that of life itself. Some visualize an impending illness followed shortly by death, others foresee a brief period of good health preceding a long and miserable decline, and many are aware of the likelihood of many years of good health and fruitful existence; still, most perceive almost tangibly that they may not live as long as they once expected to, and they suddenly feel the psychic weight which the threat of grave illness brings.

There can be a powerful sense of loss surrounding thoughts about children: parents wonder if they will have the opportunity to see their children grow up, and patients who have not yet had children but wish to do so can feel that there is no longer any hope that they will. Romance is affected as well. People in committed relationships sometimes anticipate rejection by their partner(s), while others feel as though they have lost the possibility of finding one. In either case they envision a loss of romantic companionship, which is both painful and frightening. Those who believe that their relationships will continue, or who can imagine themselves dating and seeking involvements, often mourn the loss of spontaneity and carefree intimacy implied by the need for safer sex practices. This prospect is not nearly so burdensome for people who have already become accustomed to risk reduction in sexual activities.

It is not unusual for the patient to visualize, and even experience, the loss of family, friends, and/or career at this point. This seems to be predicated on one of two assumptions: that the family members, friends, or co-workers will have to be told and will respond with rejection, or that the act of withholding this information, and the feelings this provokes, will place distance between people who were previously close. The expectation of loss of career can also stem from the picture of shortened life expectancy, frequent trips to the doctor, and impending illness which is still foremost in the imagination. Perhaps most comprehensive in this early process is the loss of feeling in control of one's life. Many patients seem to reach a point at which the import of all of these essential themes coalesces into the overwhelming impression that their lives are no longer their own, and that from that point on, this one event, this single test result, is going to dominate every facet of their existence.

Beyond Grief

Issues of blame and guilt tend to surface quite early. People who have engaged in behaviors which they know to carry a high risk for HIV infection may feel that they have brought it on themselves. Even when they have taken most or all of the appropriate precautions, many internalized judgmental feelings will come to the fore. Gay and bisexual men encounter their own homophobic feelings; IVDUs, heterosexuals with many sex partners, and heterosexuals whose partners are at increased risk all encounter within themselves negative societal values about their risks, and they often embrace them. Members of racial and ethnic minorities can also incorporate negative attitudes toward their groups into these feelings of culpability.

Blame is directed toward a variety of other targets as well. Partners or other sexual contacts frequently draw anger and resentment. In transfusion-related infections, the blood product recipient may blame the physician who ordered the transfusion, the hospital in which it was performed, the blood bank that processed the blood, and the blood donor. IVDUs who rarely share needles may blame the handful of needle-sharing contacts. In a more general sense, and regardless of the nature of the risk, fate (or God) is often the object of anger for unfairly singling out the individual to be infected.

When the test has been performed in relation to an altruistic activity, such as volunteering for the Peace Corps, travel to foreign countries for relief or missionary work, or blood donation, the giving spirit which motivated them is seen as being responsible for the ensuing delivery of what they feel to be very bad news. The seropositivity seems to be a dreadfully unjust retribution for the kindest of intentions. In a similar manner, the clinician can be the object of anger and resentment as the messenger bearing the test result, especially if he or she was the person who suggested that the test be done.

The Medical Context

A positive HIV antibody test takes on a unique significance when it serves to establish or confirm a medical diagnosis. This is the case when a patient has a clinical picture which is consistent with the effects of HIV infection, but which might be due to other causes. In these situations the findings are not sufficient to indicate with certainty a diagnosis of AIDS or active HIV-related disease, but when they are corroborated by the positive test result, a knowledgeable clinician is able to make the diagnosis of "ARC"* or AIDS (Barnes 1988). Now, the bulk of literature addressing post-test counseling presupposes that the person being tested has no symptoms, or mild ones at most, and much of the counseling focuses on the fact that being seropositive does not mean that the person has AIDS, nor that the person is ill in any way. Many of the fears arising from the test result are addressed by directing attention to the present state of good health, and to the various ways in which one can attempt to prevent or postpone the development of illness. Typical of educational materials for people being tested is the statement that "a positive test by itself does not mean that you have AIDS" (New York City Department of Health 1988). Such materials are not relevant to the situation where the patient *does* have AIDS or ARC, and may prove confusing and distressing if accidentally given to the patient whose diagnosis has been established by the test. In these circumstances the traditional discussions about incubation periods (the interval of time between infection and the development of symptoms) do not apply, although education about preventing transmission of HIV is as important as ever. The emphasis therefore shifts from trying to defer a remote and

---

*ARC is an informal diagnosis, and refers to illness caused by HIV but not conforming to the definition of AIDS.

theoretical onset of symptoms to efforts to preserve (or possibly restore) a damaged immune system, treat the present manifestations of disease, and avoid preventable complications. The presence of active HIV disease also brings the prospect of death much closer than it might be if there were no signs of damage to the immune system. Although therapies for HIV infection and its complications continue to improve, and the course which any one person will experience cannot be predicted with accuracy, there is ample evidence that most people presently diagnosed with AIDS have markedly shortened life expectancy, and many cannot expect to live more than a few years after diagnosis (Centers for Disease Control 1989). This may force both clinician and patient to deal with issues of death and dying at a much earlier point than in other testing situations.

All of the reactions that accompany a positive test result in the asymptomatic (healthy) patient may also be seen in the context of an ARC or AIDS diagnosis. Being ill raises additional concerns because, unlike being seropositive without symptoms, it is much harder to conceal from one's co-workers, household, and family. For people whose risk behavior carries a social stigma, such as male homosexual activity or IV drug use, the advent of illness may force a "coming out of the closet" of both the risk factor and the diagnosis at the same time. This is usually a traumatic experience for everyone involved, and the prospect of going through it can be daunting. Concerns about career and employment also become more immediate because absences from work (for doctor's visits or illness) will have to be explained; health, life, and disability insurance in force may or may not be adequate, and the ability to continue to perform some physically demanding jobs in the future might be questioned.

Despite these additional considerations there can also be favorable reactions to the test result that signifies an ARC or AIDS diagnosis, similar to those seen with some asymptomatics. Such a diagnosis can qualify the patient for support services which would otherwise not be available; in areas of the country where there are large numbers of HIV-infected people, some service organizations must restrict eligibility on the basis of documented illness in order to conserve their resources. Concrete benefits, such as financial support for rent, food, and medical bills, may only come with a positive diagnosis. For the person who has already suffered some disability, this assistance can be extremely welcome. Also, the clarification of the cause of the symptoms, and the identification as a "person with ARC" or a "person with AIDS" (PWARC or PWA) may actually allow the patient to move ahead with life, seek new peer groups and activities, and reformulate his or her self-concept to function more productively and

happily in the new role. The action-oriented individual may be gratified by the additional opportunities for standard and experimental
medical intervention which are available to people with active HIV
disease. These tend to contrast with the more passive and supportive
approaches which are generally offered to healthy seropositives.

Decisions

At the time of notification there are a number of decisions which the
patient must contemplate. Most often the first of these is whom to tell.
Post-test counseling routinely includes cautions regarding the casual
sharing of this information, as well as strong encouragement to notify
the present and past sexual or needle-sharing contacts. The importance of informing one's health care providers is also stressed. Pru-
dence in disclosing a positive HIV antibody test result (or even the fact
of having been tested) is clearly warranted, since such disclosure
carries the very real danger of discrimination in employment, housing, health care, and insurance, and the potential loss of these. While
some of these discriminatory practices are prohibited by laws or regulations, the remedies may come too late or be sought only at great
cost. Social stigma and ostracism are also common results when this
information "gets out." Nonetheless, it is important to have one or
more confidants in one's support system with whom to share the
news and its accompanying concerns. The need to have someone to
talk with must be balanced against the possibility of rejection, which
can be emotionally devastating. Such rejection has the potential for
disaster when the result is being cut off from financial support or
being forced to leave the house.

Notifying one's contacts who are at risk for HIV infection—a
complex and sensitive issue—is vitally important. The decision of
how and when to do so touches on most of the reactions to, and
concerns about, seropositivity. Helping the patient to understand the
necessity of alerting contacts to their risk, and facilitating the development of strategies for overcoming the difficulties involved, is one of
the most challenging aspects of post-test counseling.

The issue of medical evaluation and intervention must be considered in both healthy and symptomatic seropositives. A growing number of tools exist for evaluating the immune status of the infected
individual, and a widening range of options for standard and experimental treatments that must be explored (Henry, Thurn, and Anderson 1989). A thorough medical history and physical examination,
along with appropriate baseline laboratory tests, is the minimum that
should be recommended for anyone who is seropositive, but to some

individuals this is not a welcome prospect. To them, what would be considered the most basic measure by a medical clinician represents an admission of illness, or even just an acknowledgment of the test result, and so appears unacceptable. Others may be eager to obtain evaluation but may defer any interventions indicated by the assessment, for essentially the same reasons.

Individuals who are willing to become involved with service organizations or support groups are generally provided with a wider range of information, which can make these decisions and many others much easier to approach. A significant degree of comfort with one's seropositivity is required before such a step can be taken, and this is rarely the case in the time immediately following notification.

Delayed Reactions

A single office visit usually does not offer enough time to provide post-test counseling and carry out medical evaluation, so follow-up visits are advisable. When seropositives are seen 1 or 2 weeks after receiving their positive test results, they are likely to report some combination of common responses: varying degrees of sleeplessness, anger, sadness, and anxiety are experienced individually, or together as in depression. The majority describe an exaggerated and unrealistic concern about infecting those around them; despite the intellectual knowledge that HIV is not transmitted casually (Francis and Chin 1987) they relate that they will not allow others to drink from their glass or kiss them on the lips. Some will even refrain from touching other people, with the thought that nobody would knowingly wish to touch someone who was infected with HIV. This naturally adds to the sense of isolation that arises from feeling unable to talk about what is upsetting them.

Hypochondriacal reactions are frequently seen, as are sexual dysfunction or loss of interest in sexual activity. People who had not previously thought of themselves as being at risk for HIV infection commonly report a heightened sensitivity to any mention of AIDS and HIV in the media, as well as "AIDS jokes" and comments. Some of those inclined toward chemical dependency resume or increase their drug/alcohol use, while a few attempt to abruptly stop the use of all drugs, including tobacco, as a dramatic gesture toward health maintenance. Involvement with religion is often renewed or strengthened, as may occur with any situation that is perceived to be life-threatening.

Once again, denial of part or all of the significance of seropositivity sometimes persists. The patient requests multiple repetitions of the test, refuses further evaluation, is reticent in discussing the results of the test or any feelings about it, and occasionally just "disappears" and attempts to avoid contact with anyone who might serve as a reminder of the test result. In the opposite situation the patient becomes dependent on the medical care provider for counseling and emotional support. While such support has a place in the delivery of patient care, most medical clinicians have neither the time nor the expertise to provide the appropriate level of counseling required in these cases. It is therefore advisable to help the patient understand the benefits of seeing a mental health professional who has the training, experience, and time to be of the greatest help. It can be useful to point out that effective stress management is an essential component of medical care and health maintenance, and that competent counseling or psychotherapy may be the best "prescription" for starting such a program (Mount 1986).

THE INCONCLUSIVE TEST RESULT

As mentioned previously, HIV antibody testing occasionally produces an inconclusive or "indeterminate" test result, which means that it is neither positive nor negative. The interpretation is based on the specific details of the result, the patient's medical history, and an accurate history of activities that might have resulted in HIV infection. The inconclusive result can be more distressing than a positive one, because it means that the test will have to be repeated 1 or more months later, and that 6 or more months may pass before an accurate interpretation can be made. This emotional "limbo" tends to hinder the resolution of conflicts and development of coping mechanisms which would otherwise begin soon after learning of seropositivity. As long as a question remains, the patient does not feel as if it is permissible to process the possibility of a positive result. There follows a sense of anxiety and upset without a clear mode of resolution. This is particularly true when the clinician cannot offer any opinion about the likely outcome of future tests. If the possibility of infection is remote, and the indeterminate result is felt to be due to biological factors unrelated to HIV, the level of anxiety is usually much lower. When there is information to suggest that the result is due to recent infection, and that future tests are likely to be positive, such optimism is rarely seen. Still, there are those who tenaciously cling to the hope that everything will come out "all right," and are content to accept any degree of uncertainty in place of the fact of a positive result.

THE NEGATIVE TEST RESULT

Medical clinicians are often no less pleased than their patients when the result is negative, and there is generally a pronounced sense of relief when the result is given. Such relief is properly moderated by caution whenever testing is done shortly after an episode which might have resulted in HIV transmission (i.e., unprotected sexual intercourse). The reassurance offered by the test must presuppose follow-up testing in 6 to 12 months and the absolute avoidance of risky activities in the interim.

Feelings of invulnerability may also result; an individual who has practiced high-risk activities sometimes feels immune to infection after testing negative. This false and dangerous assumption warrants exploration, and the safer, more realistic attitude that such good fortune is not likely to last should be encouraged.

CONCLUSION

In delivering HIV antibody test results to a patient the medical care provider is dealing with an explosive combination of issues. The implications span such wide-ranging topics as sexuality, health, religion, science, bigotry, chemical dependency, love, hope, family, friendship, and death. Most medical clinicians have little academic training for handling such situations, but we can prepare ourselves by becoming familiar with the common reactions patients may have, and some of the reasons for them. We can examine our own feelings, biases, and limitations. Some of the most effective preparation comes from asking ourselves how various reactions might make us feel, and what expressions of emotion make us anxious. Which risk behaviors do we make judgments about (which activities do we think are "bad," or that people should just not do them?). Are we comfortable having an open and direct discussion about death, or about specific sexual practices? How will we respond when patients make choices which we do not recommend?

By anticipating patients' responses, and our own, we can create strategies that allow us to be most effective in our post-test counseling. For example, the awareness of "normal" reactions enables us to reassure patients that what they are experiencing is to be expected, and something that will be worked through in time (a very productive intervention). Consequently, by understanding the components of the crisis that may arise when we reveal a test result, we are able to develop resources to assist our patients in the formidable task of redefining themselves, establishing new plans, and keeping or regaining control of their lives.

REFERENCES

American Blood Commission Task Force on AIDS. 1985. Public Education: Facts about the use of the HTLV-III antibody test at blood and plasma collection facilities. In syllabus of *AIDS: Ethics and the Blood Supply* (conference), Arlington, VA, 6.

Barnes, D.M. 1988. Losing AIDS antibodies. *Science* 240:3.

Centers for Disease Control. 1989. AIDS and case-fatality rates by half-year of diagnosis, United States. *AIDS Weekly Surveillance Report—United States*, February 13:4.

Centers for Disease Control. 1988. Update: Serologic testing for antibody to human immunodeficiency virus. *Morbid. Mortal. Weekly Rep.* 36:839

Centers for Disease Control. 1987. Public Health Service guidelines for counseling and antibody testing to prevent HIV infection and AIDS. *Morbid. Mortal. Weekly Rep.* 361:509.

Centers for Disease Control. 1987. Revision of the CDC surveillance case definition for acquired immunodeficiency syndrome. *Morbid. Mortal. Weekly Rep.* 36(1S):4S–7S.

Francis, D.P., Chin, J. 1987. The prevention of acquired immunodeficiency syndrome in the United States. *J.A.M.A.* 257:1358–59.

Henry, K., Thurn, J., Anderson, D. 1989. Testing for human immunodeficiency virus: what to do if the result is positive. *Postgrad. Med.* 85 (1):301–309.

Mount, B.M. 1986. Dealing with our losses. *J. Clin. Oncology* 4:1127–1134.

New York City Department of Health. 1988. *You Have Been Told That You Are H.I.V. Antibody. . . . Positive.* Post-test information pamphlet.

Wilber, J. 1988. Research methods for studying HIV infection. *Focus* 3 (12):3.

ADDITIONAL READING

Focus: A Guide to AIDS Research and Counseling (current and back issues). UCSF AIDS Health Project, Box 0884, San Francisco CA 94943.

Morrisett, W. R. 1988. HIV antibody counseling and testing. *Physician Assistant* 12(11):96–104.

3

Positive and Negative Effects of HIV Antibody Screening

Tony W. Cheung, MD, FACP, and Fred Rosner, MD, FACP

The acquired immunodeficiency syndrome (AIDS) was first described in 1981 (Hymes, Cheung, Greene, et al. 1981). The etiological viral agent was discovered in 1983 by French scientists led by Dr. Luc Montagnier (Barre-Sinoussi, Nugeyre, Dauguet, et al. 1983). The AIDS virus is now called the human immundeficiency virus (HIV). In 1984, a serological test to detect the presence of the virus became available for research. On March 2, 1985, HIV antibody tests were licensed by the Food and Drug Administration (FDA) for testing donated units of blood and plasma.

Since 1985, the use of HIV antibody testing has increased among certain high risk and other individuals. The Public Health Service has published a series of recommendations for counseling and antibody testing to prevent HIV infection and AIDS (Centers for Disease Control 1987). Certain groups, such as the U.S. military, advocate broad-based screening of large populations (or even of the entire population) to detect persons who are infected. This chapter reviews the basis of screening for HIV infection and examines the positive and negative effects of HIV screening and testing programs.

PRINCIPLES OF SCREENING FOR MEDICAL DISORDERS INCLUDING HIV

It is important to distinguish between "screening" and "testing." "Screening" is the application of HIV antibody tests to a population of persons who are generally healthy or asymptomatic. Persons who have a positive screening test are referred for or provided with more definitive diagnostic procedures for confirmation of the test results. By contrast, "testing" is the application of tests or procedures to individuals on a case-by-case basis.

HIV antibody screening may be voluntary or mandatory, may be applied systematically or nonuniformly, and may involve entire populations or only selected target populations. Few screening programs have been implemented nationally, or even statewide, although some programs involve large populations in certain target areas. Participation in most screening programs is voluntary; only a few, such as the screening of newborns for phenylketonuria and hypothyroidism, are required by law.

Currently, all donated blood is tested for HIV antibodies. Mandatory HIV testing is also required for foreign service employees; blood, organ, or sperm donors; military personnel; immigrants; and inmates in federal prisons. In Illinois and Louisiana testing is required for marriage licenses.

In general, most screening programs provide a specific benefit for the person being screened. Some programs screen for early diagnosis of a condition amenable to definitive therapy, such as cervical carcinoma in situ (pap smear), syphilis, or tuberculosis. Other programs screen to provide improved therapy and management of a chronic condition such as hypertension or diabetes mellitus. Some screening programs provide information about the carrier status of a genetic disease. Most screening programs are conducted in conjunction with health care delivery. Screening for certain abnormalities such as HIV infection may produce serious psychological effects on the person, potentially create discrimination if confidentiality is not maintained, and potentially cause social disruption because of the panic and fear engendered by the AIDS epidemic.

ETHICAL CONSIDERATIONS

HIV antibody screening can produce both positive and negative effects on society. It is therefore important to evaluate any screening program from an ethical viewpoint and to consider "respect for persons," the "harm" principle (limitations on an individual's liberty to pursue goals that will harm others), "beneficence" (acting on behalf of the interests and welfare of others), and "justice" (fair distribution of benefits and burdens). Based on these ethical considerations, Bayer and co-workers established seven prerequisites for ethical screening programs (Bayer, Levine, and Wolf 1986):

1. The purpose of the screening must be ethically acceptable.
2. The means to be used in the screening program and the intended use of the information must be appropriate for accomplishing the purpose.

3. High-quality laboratory services must be used.
4. Individuals must be notified that screening will take place.
5. Individuals who are screened have a right to be informed about the results.
6. Sensitive and supportive counseling programs must be available before and after screening to interpret the results, whether they are positive or negative.
7. The confidentiality of screened individuals must be protected.

Although these ethical principles may at times conflict with each other, (e.g., protecting the public health versus respecting the autonomy and privacy of persons), these principles "constitute the threshold requirements for ethical acceptability" of screening programs. Moreover, the positive effects of a screening program can only come about if these ethical prerequisites are built into the program.

POSITIVE EFFECTS OF SCREENING

Since there is no cure for AIDS, the best way to contain the disease is presently by prevention through education. An essential goal for the HIV screening program is to control the spread of the disease. Screening blood donors eliminates transmission from that source, since HIV positive blood and its components are not used for transfusion. Likewise, contaminated organs and sperm are not used. Prior to the initiation of HIV screening of donated blood and plasma in the spring of 1985, the HIV seroprevalence rate among blood donors ranged from 0.01% to 0.2%. With HIV antibody screening of all donated blood, heat treatment of clotting factor concentrates to kill the virus, and the elimination of blood donation from high risk individuals, HIV transmission by blood and blood products has been practically eliminated.

Education is a very important tool in reducing HIV transmission. HIV testing provides an excellent opportunity for the physician or counselor to educate and offer advice to the client or patient with respect to HIV infection. Such education is an important part of pretest counseling and serves to help prevent the transmission of HIV. Effective counseling is essential to the success of the HIV antibody blood testing procedure. The counseling and educational process provides information about the virus, the diseases it produces, routes of transmission, and methods of reducing risk.

Since persons who are HIV antibody positive are capable of transmitting their infection to others, such HIV-infected persons need to be educated about their lifestyles and told about changes necessary to prevent infecting others. The basis of good education and counseling begins with an accurate medical history, including sexual and drug use history. A client reluctant to give accurate information about risk behavior poses a serious problem for the counselor trying to offer advice on risk reduction. The best circumstance is when the client expresses interest in obtaining information on AIDS or the HIV antibody test. Using frank, non-judgmental, open-ended questions in history taking, the counselor can determine whether a client is at risk for exposure to or transmission of HIV. Using this information, the counselor can offer the correct advice to his client about behavior alteration. A homosexual man might be informed about "safer" sex by the use of condoms and monogamy; an intravenous (IV) drug user would be strongly encouraged to enter a drug detoxification program and avoid heterosexual relationships without "protected sex." Persons who are at risk, but test HIV antibody negative also require education about how to avoid becoming infected. Thus, testing persons for the HIV antibody through screening programs becomes a method to target specific educational and counseling programs to induce behavior changes in life-styles that minimize or eliminate the risk of HIV infection and transmission.

As many as 50% of the newborns of HIV-infected women can contract the disease from their mothers either transplacentally or during parturition. Therefore, all women of childbearing age who are in high risk groups should be given information about AIDS, HIV infection, and the availability of counseling and testing for the HIV antibody. Education and testing before pregnancy maximizes the choices of HIV-infected women to avoid pregnancy and subsequent intrauterine or perinatal HIV infection of their newborns.

For a pregnant client, various options, such as therapeutic termination of pregnancy, or participation in a clinical trial to learn about azidothymidine (AZT) in pregnancy, are presented to the client. The identification of HIV-positive women early in pregnancy is important to ensure appropriate medical care for the women, plan medical care for their infants, counsel about future pregnancies, and provide information about the risk of sexual transmission of HIV to others.

Knowledge about HIV infection is important for health and personal planning on the part of society, as well as the HIV-positive person. From the public health perspective, effective interventions in the current AIDS epidemic lie in the development of thorough serological screening studies to examine changes in HIV prevalence and behavioral patterns of high risk persons and the general population.

From an individual perspective, knowing one's HIV antibody status permits the person's health professionals to make the necessary plans for health care, and to request social services (including counseling) where needed. Early recognition of HIV infection allows the physician to monitor the client's immunologic and neurologic status, and to prescribe prophylactive therapy against opportunistic infections such as *Pneumocystis carinii* pneumonia and tuberculosis. Live viral vaccines should not be given to an HIV-positive person because of the danger of developing disseminated infections such as vaccinia. Further, a positive serologic history of HIV exposure allows the physician to increase his index of suspicion in recognizing the early onset of opportunistic infections and other AIDS-related signs and symptoms, so that timely diagnosis and treatment can be implemented. Such efforts can result in a reduction of the case-fatality rate of patients with AIDS (Rothenberg, Woelfel, Stoneburner, et al.1987). Furthermore, these individuals can be considered for antiviral clinical trials (e.g., using AZT for asymptomatic HIV-infected persons) or take advantage of the new scientific discoveries as soon as they are made available.

Another positive effect of screening for HIV infection is that it allows one to take charge of one's future. Without knowledge of his HIV status, a person in a high risk group always faces uncertainty. Such a person may consider himself positive without even testing and alter his lifestyle or behavior because society has labeled him "positive". Knowing one's HIV antibody status removes this uncertainty. Knowing that his HIV antibody is positive allows the client to take measures to prevent transmission of the virus, seek medical attention, and plan for the unavoidable future of the full-blown illness of AIDS, including the possibility of early death. If the client is HIV-negative, he should continue behavior that will prevent him from contracting the illness, and with the anxiety of not knowing alleviated, and he can function as a "normal" person.

NEGATIVE EFFECTS OF SCREENING

Many persons who are at risk of HIV infection are concerned that the results of the screening programs may be used against them. Transmission of HIV from one person to another occurs through sexual contact (homosexual or heterosexual) or through the sharing of blood-contaminated needles during the injection of drugs. Nevertheless, there is fear among the public that has resulted in numerous suggestions about the need to control the spread of HIV by quarantining persons who are infected. If this suggestion were adopted, hemophiliac children who contracted the virus from blood products would not be allowed to return to school. Even if they were permitted to return to school, other fearful parents would take their children out of school to avoid their having contact with a classmate with AIDS.

A substantial number of Americans believe that "those with AIDS should not be allowed to live in their neighborhood or community, and they favor landlords having the right to evict those with the disease" (Blendon and Donelan 1988). In Florida, a home with children infected with the AIDS virus was set on fire by a misguided arsonist. Finding appropriate housing for persons with the virus can be a formidable task. In addition, various forms of social ostracism have been reported (Stempel, Moulton, Kelly, et al. 1987; Douglas, Harper, and Polk 1987).

Maintenance of confidentiality and respect for the patient's autonomy are essential elements of any screening program. Confidentiality encourages people to participate in the screening and to seek treatment if needed. It also protects them from adverse consequences. Since persons infected with HIV are at high risk of premature death from AIDS or associated conditions, health and life insurance companies deny insurance to new applicants or refuse to renew policies already in place (Blendon and Donelan 1988). Employers do not wish to incur expenses to train workers who may become ill and die, and therefore deny such persons job opportunities. The "domino effect" of job and insurance discrimination may reflect itself in denial of bank loans, mortgages, and other forms of credit to HIV-positive persons. The result of such discrimination may be disastrous for a young, productive member of society who is HIV positive and still asymptomatic. Therefore, it is important for physicians to protect their patients and clients by keeping confidential information from persons who might misuse such information.

Another negative aspect of HIV screening is the psychiatric disturbances which might result from learning that one is HIV positive. Goldblum and Seymour cite a variety of such symptoms, including "severe anxiety, depression, suicidal ideation, intrusive thoughts, nightmares, and sleep disturbances," as well as "interpersonal problems ranging from blaming the partner and sexual dysfunction to homicidal rage" (Goldblum and Seymour 1987). Learning that one is seropositive for HIV antibody is profoundly distressing, even among people who anticipate a positive outcome of the test in advance. They may react with expressions of disbelief, anger, fear, guilt, or self-recrimination (Wilkie 1987). Most feel a sense of hopelessness and helplessness in the first few weeks. An anxiety complex which may include agitation, panic attacks, anorexia, tachycardia, and insomnia, as well as clinical depression, may also be noted (Faulstich 1987; Miller

1987). Some HIV-positive persons may have suicidal thoughts and think they already have AIDS, are going to die, and are therefore in a medical crisis (Marzuk, Tierney, Tardiff, et al. 1988).

Most HIV-infected women are of childbearing age and should be made to understand that they can transmit the infection to their babies before or during birth, or while breastfeeding. Limitations on childbearing can cause extreme distress in both men and women. Seropositive individuals may encounter problems in their sexual relationships because of their potential to infect others. Moreover, people who are HIV positive often struggle with lowered self-esteem and social isolation, which may or may not be self-inflicted. They may withdraw from people who are important to them for fear of infecting them—even through casual contact. Self-destructive behavior tends to be common in AIDS patients with personality disorders (Holland and Tross 1985).

It is prudent for counselors to identify the psychosocial backgrounds of their clients. Counselors should correct their client's misunderstandings and seek the necessary support system for their clients. Clients should be encouraged to meet with self-help groups or other individuals to share their concerns and learn better ways of coping with stress.

There is a similarity between the panic experienced by HIV seropositive individuals about whether or not they will develop AIDS and the fear of cancer patients in anticipating recurrence of disease or metastases (Weisman and Worden 1976, 1977; Morin, Charles, and Malyon 1984). The rate of conversion from seropositive status to AIDS is from 10% to 50% within 5 years (Curran, Jaffe, Hardy, et al.1988). Such information has greatly increased the level of anxiety. Therefore, like cancer patients, HIV-positive persons need help to retain hope about their health and about scientific progress to prevent the progression of, and find a cure for, the disease. Such clients also need continuing reassurance, support, and access to good health care to maintain an optimal degree of functioning and to avoid the excessive anxiety that could result in destructive behavior.

Persons who are seronegative obviously feel tremendously relieved, but may have a false sense of security. If they were exposed to the virus within the previous 6 to 12 weeks, they may not yet have developed detectable antibodies. Some high-risk individuals who test negative may conclude that they must be immune to HIV infection, and therefore believe that they can engage in high-risk behavior with impunity (Wilkie 1987).

Lastly, the cost of mandatory or universal HIV screening is high and might lead to reduced funding of other important medical and social needs. Decisions about instituting mandatory testing for HIV antibody (e.g. premarital testing) can be based in part on the cost-effectiveness in terms of preventing further spread of HIV infection, taking into account area prevalence and other factors. Most persons in the U.S. are at low risk of infection. The prevalence of infection among highly selected populations of blood donors is only a few per 10,000, while among persons seeking marriage licenses it is estimated to be less than 1 per 10,000 (Schorr, Berkowitz, Cumming, et al. 1985). Therefore, screening the entire population to detect a few persons who are infected is not likely to be cost-effective.

REFERENCES

Barre-Sinoussi F., M. Nugeyre, C. Dauguet, et al. 1983. Isolation of a T-lymphotropic retrovirus from a patient at risk for acquired immune deficiency syndrome. *Science.* 220:868-871.

Bayer R., C. Levine, and S.M. Wolf. 1986. HIV antibody screening—an ethical framework for evaluating proposed programs. *J.A.M.A.* 256:1768-1774.

Blendon R.J., and K. Donelan 1988. Discriminating against people with AIDS. *N. Engl. J. Med.* 319:1022-1026.

Centers for Disease Control. 1987. Public Health Service Guidelines for counseling and antibody testing to prevent HIV infection and AIDS. *Morbid. Mortal. Weekly Rep.* 36:509-515.

Coates T., S. Morin, and L. McKusick 1986. The psychological and behavioral consequences of AIDS antibody testing. Presented at the National Institute of Health AIDS Methodology Conference, Bethesda, MD.

Curran J.W., H.W. Jaffe, A.M. Hardy, et al. 1988. Epidemiology of HIV infection and AIDS in the United States. *Science*, 239:610-161.

Douglas D.K., M. Harper, and F. Polk. 1987. HIV positivity: The psychosocial impact of donor notification. Presented at the Third International Conference on AIDS, Washington, DC.

Faulstich M.E. 1987. Psychiatric aspects of AIDS. *Am. J. Psychiatry* 144:551-556.

Gallo R., S. Salahuddin, M. Popvic, et al. 1984. Frequent detection and isolation of cytopathic retrovirus (HTLV-III) from patients with AIDS and at risk for AIDS. *Science* 224:500-503.

Goldblum P. and N. Seymour. 1987. Whether to take the test: counseling guidelines. *Focus—A Guide to AIDS Research* 2:1.

Holland J.C. and S. Tross. 1985. The psychosocial and neuropsychiatric sequelae of the immunodeficiency syndrome and related disorders. *Ann. Intern. Med.* 103:760-764.

Hymes K., T. Cheung, J.B. Greene, et al. 1981. Kaposi's sarcoma in homosexual men. *Lancet* 2:598-600.

Marzuk P.M., H. Tierney, K. Tardiff, et al. 1988. Increased risk of suicide in persons with AIDS. *J.A.M.A.* 259:1333-1337.

Miller D. 1987. HIV Counseling: Some practical problems and issues. *J. Royal Soc. Med.* 80:278-280.

Morin S.F., K.A. Charles, and A.K. Malyon. 1984. The psychological impact of AIDS on gay men. *Am. Psychologist* 39:1288-1293.

New York Times, September 30, 1985.

Rothenberg R., M. Woelfel, R. Stoneburner, et al. 1987. Survival with the AIDS experience with 5,833 cases in New York City. *N. Eng. J. Med.*, 317:1297-1302.

Schorr J.B., A. Berkowitz, P.D. Cumming, et al. 1985. Prevalence of HTLV-III antibody in American blood donors (letter). *N. Eng. J. Med.* 313:384-385.

Siegal F.P., C. Lopez, G.S. Hammer, et al. 1981. Severe acquired immunodeficiency in male homosexuals, manifested by chronic perianal ulcerative herpes simplex lesions. *N. Eng. J. Med.* 305:1439-1444.

Stempel R., J. Moulton, T. Kelly, et al. 1987. Patterns of distress following HIV antibody test notification. Presented at the Third International Conference on AIDS, Washington,DC.

Weisman A., and W. Worden. 1976, 1977. The existential plight in cancer: significance of the first 100 days. *Int. J. Psychiatric Med.*, 7:1-15.

Wilkie P.A. 1987. Counseling in HIV infection. *Scot. Med. J.* 32:114-116.

4

Ethics and AIDS

Judith Grad, JD

The ethical questions surrounding HIV infection are many and difficult. Let us begin with the ethical problems and responsibilities of the central person, the seropositive-for-HIV person (a "Positive" for the purposes of this chapter) or possible Positive.

ETHICS ISSUES FOR THE INDIVIDUAL

Voluntary Testing

There are two basic reasons for a person to want to be tested for HIV, both of great personal importance, and one a serious ethical obligation. First, there is the person's own health. Treatments have been and are being developed that can delay the onset of ARC or AIDS, and improve the quality and duration of life if AIDS does develop (Gay Men's Health Crisis). Second, from the moment a person is infected with HIV he is capable of transmitting it, to his sexual partners and, if he is an intravenous (IV) drug user to those with whom he shares needles. If he has the infection and doesn't know it, he may be endangering the lives and health of others.

People fear testing for various reasons. They are not sure they can emotionally handle a positive result, or they fear that the information will "get out" and they will be discriminated against (Gay Men's Health Crisis). In many places, great care is taken to keep the information confidential. Sometimes, as in New York, confidentiality is required by law (Laws of New York 1988). It is a good idea for a person who thinks he could be positive to seek counseling or therapy before he takes the test as well as when he gets the results (Gay Men's Health Crisis).

In my opinion, a person who thinks he may be at risk and who is engaging (or may engage) in activities which would put others at risk, is morally obligated either to establish that he is seronegative or to refrain from such activities. A person who may be at risk and has tested seronegative should nevertheless practice safer sex (Gay Men's Health Crisis) not only for his own protection, but also because he has a moral obligation to those whom he might infect. The usual screening test ("enzyme-linked immunosorbent assay"—ELISA) detects antibodies to the virus rather than the virus itself, and if the test was taken after he was infected but before he developed antibodies (which could take up to 3 years), or if he became infected after the test, the negative result would be incorrect. There is a new technique called "polymerase chain reaction" which detects the virus itself, including virus hidden in cells. This test, according to the *New York Times* (June 1, 1989), is available in only two laboratories in the U.S. and is costly. High-risk people who have taken only the ELISA test and have had a negative result should behave, in terms of the ethical responsibility not to infect other people, as though they may be infected, as indeed they may. Such a person, like someone who has tested positive, is obviously morally obligated not to donate blood.

The ethical obligation of an IV drug abuser who has been sharing needles and tests positive are all those listed above and below, plus getting into a drug program and off drugs as soon as possible. He would probably be deluding himself if he resolved to continue with the drugs, but never again share somebody's needle or works. Being high impairs both judgment and resolution.

Disclosure

If a person tests seropositive, the next ethical question to be faced is who he is obligated to tell. The confidentiality laws apply to other people, not to the Positive. He may tell anyone. It should go without saying, but cannot go without saying, that a spouse or any other sexual partner (or partners) must be told. Even if the Positive is practicing safer sex, the risk of transmitting the virus, while greatly reduced, is not eliminated. If the partner is willing to take that reduced risk, he or she is free to do so, but it must be the partner's knowing choice. Many in the gay community (and perhaps elsewhere) are convinced that the practice of safer sex eliminates the need to disclose. I cannot agree. As to past partners, they have a right to know that they may have been infected so that they can take whatever steps are indicated.

Since HIV is not communicated by ordinary contact, there is ordinarily no obligation to tell such people as relatives, landlords, employers, or platonic friends. Telling them, or not, is the Positive's own choice.

A major factor to be considered in balancing the patient's right to confidentiality with the rights of others to know that he is positive, is dementia. When we think of an HIV-infected surgeon, for example, we think of all that blood (although it is generally the patient's blood, not the surgeon's), and we imagine his patient coming down with AIDS years later, and eventually dying. The real danger is that the surgeon may develop dementia as his first symptom of full-blown AIDS, make a mistake in the surgery, and lose his patient right there on the table. Dementia occurs in many AIDS patients, is sometimes the first symptom, and is the result of direct neurological impairment caused by the virus rather than an opportunistic infection. It can begin insidiously, with loss of recent memory, impairment of judgment and, sometimes, belligerence.

When is the surgeon, the lawyer, the motorman, or anyone else whose judgment significantly affects other people, ethically obligated to give up his work? To what extent is the Positive's employer, patient, or client entitled to know that the Positive is in danger of becoming demented? Much thought and study will be needed to provide even partial answers to these questions because a Positive may go on for years without developing AIDS, and could have AIDS for some time without dementia. This issue is an example of the tensions between the public good and individual liberties (Levine 1986).

Pregnancy

Suppose a woman's HIV test and her pregnancy test both come out positive at the same time. She is then faced with a question that has two clear, unambiguous, and totally opposite ethical answers. There is a 30% to 65% chance that if a baby is born to her, it will be born with HIV infection acquired either in utero or during the birth process (Gay Men's Health Crisis). There is also a very high probability that the child will not reach maturity with a living mother.

Some people believe, as I do, that it is morally wrong to risk bearing a child who has so high a likelihood of living a short life that will end in excruciating pain. One counselor who was not expected to advise clients as to whether or not to abort was reported to ask every pregnant Positive: "Have you ever heard an AIDS baby cry?" Such people would choose abortion of the fetus. If pregnancy has not yet occurred when a woman discovers she is positive, pregnancy should of course be avoided. Some women might even feel, although this has not been much discussed, that they must choose between celibacy and sterilization, even if they practice safer sex in an effort to protect their partners.

Others, on religious or other grounds, believe that it is always morally wrong to abort a fetus, considering it equivalent to murder. Catholics are not alone in preaching this doctrine. It is taught by

Orthodox Jews and Muslims, many evangelical Protestants, and some black preachers, who hold that abortion is genocide.

The choice is difficult for many women. Sometimes, when the Positive woman is a drug abuser no choice is made until she delivers, then abandons the infant. If the child is infected, finding a home where he can be cared for, and with luck, loved, is extremely difficult.

HEALTH PROVIDERS

The AIDS epidemic has provoked considerable discussion and controversy about medical ethics in many areas.

Refusal to Treat

The extent of a physician's obligation to treat varies widely according to who you ask (Volberding and Abrams 1985). In practice, the willingness or refusal of a physician to treat a Positive depends more on what pressures can be applied than on his personal version of medical ethics. It is generally believed among doctors that if a patient of long-standing becomes HIV-infected, his doctor has an ethical obligation to continue treating him (unless the particular treatment required is outside his area of competence), but that he is free to refuse a prospective new patient who is infected (Arras 1988).

For many years the physician's risk of infection was not a major issue because practicing medicine was no longer considered, with modern control of disease transmission and cure, to be dangerous. By contrast, in centuries gone by many physicians refused to treat plague victims and fled plague areas. When the existence of AIDS became known, a panic ensued that is equivalent to the medieval fear of the plague, not only among laypersons (Kübler-Ross 1987), but also among those in the health-providing community. Although the risk that a health worker will become infected by HIV, even if exposed (e.g., stuck by a contaminated needle), is really quite small (Allen 1988), many doctors, dentists, and other health providers decided that it was a risk they were not willing to take. For many, especially those with ARC or full-blown AIDS, treatment is mainly available from those who are compelled to render it, such as interns and residents in hospitals that depend on government funds (Volberding and Abrams 1985). Now that the size of the risk is becoming known, the panic reaction may diminish in the medical community, and for more and more providers, ethics will outbalance fear.

For psychotherapists, the risk of becoming infected because of their work is a flat level zero. Psychotherapists do not come into contact with the bodily fluids of their patients. Therapists have usually felt free to refuse to treat persons with whom they felt so uncomfortable that the quality of treatment would be compromised, but I suggest that a therapist who is led to refuse patients because of a fear of something that cannot happen may need to look deeply into his own psyche.

Confidentiality and Compulsory Testing

The issues of confidentiality and compulsory testing are so intertwined that they are discussed together here. The main theme that connects them is the existence, extent, and intensity of discrimination against HIV carriers, and sometimes against their families and associates as well (Kübler-Ross 1987). People known to be positive, even if asymptomatic, have lost jobs, apartments, educational opportunities, and even access to health care because of the fear of AIDS.

Because compulsory testing is ordinarily for the purpose of informing some person or institution (other than the person to be tested) of the results, some confidentiality is by definition lost, and the fear that the information will be further communicated by the entity for whom the test was made is far from unreasonable, even though public health authorities generally have a good reputation for maintaining confidentiality. Thus, the public health and other values of compulsory testing and disclosure must be balanced against the individual's rights, constitutional or otherwise, to be protected from discrimination. The gay community and others have vigorously and sometimes successfully fought both compulsory testing and disclosure.

Where do the equities lie, and assuming the argument that ethics follows the equities, what is right here? Perhaps that depends on the reason for testing or disclosure. An employer who demands compulsory testing in order to help keep his insurance rates down has a harder job justifying such testing than a hospital that would test all pregnant women. Insurance companies have the power to, and sometimes do, insist on testing. The individual must choose between taking the test and foregoing the policy. It has been claimed, not without merit, that once a piece of information is on an insurance company's computers, it is no longer confidential. There may be constitutional grounds for rejecting compulsory testing, but the courts have already indicated that, if so, there will be exceptions.

Making a constitutional argument against all disclosure would be difficult. Many communicable diseases, including such sexually transmitted diseases as syphilis and gonorrhea, are required by law to be reported by physicians and other health workers to the proper public health authorities. Sexual contacts of the infected person are often informed that they have been exposed to the disease, although not necessarily by whom ("whom" may be self-evident in some situations). Such laws are not considered to violate any constitutional rights, and AIDS would seem to fit quite precisely into this legal pattern.

Even where AIDS is added to the list of reportable transmissible diseases, HIV infection without AIDS symptomatology is not, and there is some legislative and regulatory tendency toward responding to the fear of discrimination by forbidding reporting (and most other disclosure) in strong, comprehensive, and specific language. This protects the Positive from discrimination, but does not protect his past, present, and future lovers from AIDS. I refer particularly to Chapter 584 of the Laws of New York of 1988, which adds a new Article (27-F) to the Public Health Law that provides, among other things, that a person having confidential information that someone is a Positive may not disclose that information to the Positive's spouse or other sexual partner unless he is a physician. California also has confidentiality regulations. The principle embodied in the Tarasoff case (*Tarasoff* v. *Regents of the University of California* 1976) is that a psychotherapist may be held legally liable for failing to warn someone to whom his patient is a danger, if the patient inflicts the anticipated harm. In New York a non-medical psychotherapist is forbidden to give such a warning, even after having done his best to enable and persuade the patient to make the disclosure himself. One can assume that in a state where such legislation exists, the therapist is legally safe if he acts as the legislation requires, but he is placed in an ethical bind. He cannot warn the lover, even if he is convinced that the warning is ethically required, balancing the confidentiality required of therapists against the possible illness and death of the lover (Winston 1987). The state has made the choice.

Cost Containment and Proper Care

Medical ethics are primarily patient-centered (Angell 1987). A duty of the profession to society is acknowledged (Jennings 1987), but the doctor's duty to his patient is paramount. This priority was coming under considerable pressure even before the AIDS epidemic because medical care was becoming uncomfortably expensive for individuals, government, employers, insurers, and medical facilities (whose medical reimbursements received could not cover the costs of all the services they felt were required). Federal reimbursements, for example, are often standard for a particular diagnosis, without regard to the services actually rendered. A hospital can lose money by providing more or better services, or make a profit by doing less. Now that the AIDS epidemic threatens to overwhelm medical facilities and severely impact the economy, these pressures are increased. Is it a question of ethics, or public or social policy, whether PWAs should get proper medical care, even if the cost of that care damages the economy, as it is so likely to? My answer is—all of the above.

Suicide

The question of whether a physician can ethically assist a terminally ill patient to die is old, but discussion of it has become increasingly open in the presence of AIDS. According to the *New York Times* (May 24, 1989), efforts are underway in four states to make such assistance legal, but some doctors and hospitals are quietly rendering such assistance now. The question becomes acute because AIDS can cause blindness, intolerable pain, incontinence, and other indignities. Some argue that, to force a person who will soon die in any event, to endure all this any longer than he is willing to do so is wrong. Others argue that to assist suicide is always a serious violation of the physician's Hippocratic oath. The *Times* quotes a Southern Baptist minister and college teacher as having said, "The discussion has shifted. It is being discussed now not as an absolute prohibition, but as a question of under what circumstances should it be allowed."

One thing is clear. A Positive who has not yet developed AIDS, or if he has, has not progressed to a terminal stage, will not be helped by any ethical doctor to suicide at that time. A Positive is only potentially terminally ill. He may have years without any AIDS symptoms at all. If he thinks of suicide when he gets the test results, and some do, he needs counseling or therapy for living, not dying. As I recommended earlier, counseling or therapy is desirable whenever anyone takes an HIV test. Where there is depression or suicidal ideation, therapy would seem to be indicated and it is the obligation of the test administrators to recommend it.

SCIENCE AND GOVERNMENT: NEW DRUGS

After test tube and animal experiments are concluded on a potentially useful new drug, the usual scientific protocol would be based on a double-blind experiment with human subjects. This means that some of the people participating in the experiment would get the drug, while others would get a placebo, and neither the experimenters nor the subjects would know who is getting which. Scientists argue that this pattern produces valid scientific evidence, whereas giving the drug to everyone who participates destroys the validity of the experiment. AIDS patients, facing death, argue that if a drug can help them, then it should be made available to them. After the experiment is completed, and the Food and Drug Administration (FDA) has gone through its approval procedure, it may be years too late for the drug to help them. But the federal government has usually banned the distribution of untested and unapproved drugs.

Another problem with most double-blind protocols is that there are many exclusions. Women, for example, are not usually permitted to participate, because the experimenters fear that a woman may become pregnant and the experimenters would be held responsible for any damage to the fetus. It is said that a woman who could prove that she had had a tubal ligation was refused participation in an AIDS drug experiment on this ground. When large groups are excluded from testing not only does it unfairly deny those groups access to experimental drugs, but it also compromises the science. What an experiment proves to be true, for example, may be true only for white men between 22 and 30. Still, the double-blind experiment does yield more scientific information than does giving the drug to anyone who might need it and watching to see what happens. The additional information comes from comparing what happened to the people who took the drug with what happened to those who did not. An important ethical obligation in connection with such tests, procuring the informed consent of the subject, is sometimes skimped or neglected, even though federal regulations require it and many AIDS experiments are federally funded. A person who is to be the subject of such experiments must be told and must understand that although there is hope that the drug will be helpful, the purpose of the experiment is to obtain scientific information that will ultimately help many people not just to help any particular subject. He must also understand that he may or may not get the drug, and that if he does get it, it may have side effects which could be quite serious. If the proposed experimental subject has dementia, his ability to give fully informed consent could be called into question (Volberding and Abrams 1985).

It is now being argued that it is ethical and correct to give such a drug, at the physician's discretion, to persons who are not part of the experiment, since this will not affect the results of the experiment. And this is sometimes done. Under pressure, the FDA has relaxed some of its bans on allowing AIDS drugs that have not been fully tested to be distributed.

Taking or administering such drugs outside the experimental frame is a medical, not an ethical question. The extent that the government insists on going by the bureaucratic book with respect to the distribution of new AIDS drugs would be considered unethical by those who consider all unnecessary cruelty to be presumptively unethical.

REFERENCES

Allen, J.R. 1988. Health care workers and the risk of HIV transmission. *Hastings Center Rep.* (April-May): 2.
Angell, M. 1987. Medicined: the endangered patient-centered ethic. *Hastings Center Rep.* (Special Suppl.: The Public Duties of the Professions).
Arras, J.D. 1988. The fragile web of responsibility: AIDS and the duty to treat. *Hastings Center Rep.* (Special Suppl.: AIDS, the Responsibility of Health Officials).
Gay Men's Health Crisis leaflets. *Medical Answers About AIDS, The Test, An Ounce of Prevention, The Safer Sex Condom Guide.* New York: Gay Men's Health Crisis.
Jennings, B. 1987. Public interest and common good. *Hastings Center Re.* (Special Suppl.: The Public Duties of the Professions).
Kübler-Ross, E. 1987. *AIDS: The Ultimate Challenge.* New York: Macmillan.
Levine, C. 1986. Introduction. *Hastings Center Rep.* (Special Suppl.: AIDS, Public Health and Civil Liberties).
Tarasoff v. *Regents of the University of California.* 17 Cal. 3d 425, 131 Cal. Rptr. 14 (1976).
Volberding, P. and D. Abrams. 1985. Clinical care and research. *Hastings Center Rep.* (Special Suppl.: AIDS, the Emerging Ethical Dilemma).
Winston, M. 1987. Commentary: AIDS and a duty to protect. *Hastings Center Rep.* 1.

5

Is HIV Testing Desirable and Necessary?

Eulon Ross Taylor, MD and Tom McGovern, EdD

HIV testing and the outcome of such testing raise serious ethical issues. Ethics, by its nature, addresses what ought to be done in a given situation. In the matter of HIV testing, the ethical considerations must take into account the rights of the person being tested, the rights of persons who come in contact with the persons who test positive, the rights of health caregivers who care for the person, and also the public policy which we as a society institute in response to the presence of persons in our society who test positively for the virus.

The primary question which must be addressed is whether HIV testing is desirable and necessary. Some would answer "yes" to this question, some would answer "no"; another group would respond "it depends."

UTILITARIAN AND DEONTOLOGICAL APPROACHES

In determining whether or not we should be engaged in HIV testing, a number of ethical theories exist to guide us in our deliberations. Our theoretical positions give meaning to the values which guide our thinking in these areas. Some would base the argument to test or not to test and the other issues associated with testing on a cost/benefit, maximize the good and minimize the harm, utilitarian approach. Others would argue that there is some ultimate good, some ultimate sense of duty which should guide our actions. This thinking belongs to the deontological school.

It is important to ascertain which theoretical position or combination of positions guides our thinking when we approach the issue of HIV testing within an ethical framework. Typically, a utilitarian approach tends to protect the rights of the majority. Such an approach, if pushed to its ultimate limits, provides little protection or guarantee for the rights of a person testing positive for the HIV virus. On the other hand, such an approach might distribute the cost/benefit ratio of testing among the persons who are infected, those who come in contact with the person who is infected, and the rights of the society as a whole. The deontological approach, which could well appeal to some notion of ultimate justice, might dictate some ultimate sense of fairness in dealing with the many issues which surround HIV testing. Such an approach would seek to justify and maintain the dignity of all involved in such an undertaking. An appeal, however, to some ultimate source of right or wrong in this matter could well result in some strict form of moral absolutism. It might be decided that the source of the infection in some persons resulted from perceived immoral activity and as such requires condemnation rather than help or support. What is being advocated here is that we approach the theoretical basis of our ethical deliberations with some degree of caution. Our theoretical base guides and forms the principles and rules on which we base our ethical conclusions and subsequent actions.

ETHICAL PRINCIPLES

It is beyond the scope of this chapter to discuss the overall implications of the utilitarian or deontological approaches to the host of complex issues surrounding HIV testing. In the same light, it is impossible to fully articulate the application of the ethical principles of autonomy, non-maleficence, beneficence, and justice to the determination of appropriate policy and action in dealing with HIV testing. One must, however, seek to apply these principles in summary fashion to the main areas of ethical concern in the area of HIV testing. Each of these principles will be defined in a general sort of way in the introduction and then will be discussed in their relatedness or in their conflict as the various aspects of HIV testing are considered in the rest of the chapter (Beauchamp and Walter 1982).

Autonomy

Autonomy can be described as the respect for persons, a principle which guarantees the right of a competent person to self-determination, provided the rights of others are not being violated. In light of autonomy a person normally would have the right to be tested or not to be tested. Issues of informed consent would also fall under autonomy, as would the requirement of confidentiality. It is obvious that the principle of autonomy has far reaching implications for HIV testing. But what of persons whose autonomy is compromised by an impaired sense of competency or responsibility? What of persons whose drug-induced behavior or compulsive sexual behavior robs them of the self-determination necessary for responsible activity? The thorny ethical questions of applying the principle of autonomy to such individuals is obvious (Dyer 1988).

Non-maleficence

One of the oldest principles in medicine, and by implication in all other forms of health care, is the principle of non-maleficence. This principle is enshrined in the maxim *primum non nocere*, "above all, do no harm." This principle would seek to protect the individual from any harm resulting from the testing itself, as well as from testing positive. In addition, it would seek to protect non-infected individuals from being infected by the infected person and it would also seek to protect the overall good of society. The application of this principle to HIV testing is obviously difficult and complex.

Beneficence

The ethical principle of beneficence includes among its meanings the doing of good and the act of promotion of good, kindness, and charity. William Frankena (1973) writes that this principle of beneficence contains four elements: one ought not to inflict evil or harm (principle of non-maleficence), one ought to prevent evil or harm, one ought to remove evil or harm, and one ought to do or promote good. One can readily see the implications of this principle as applied within these definitions to HIV testing. Also encompassed by the principle of beneficence are the notions of competent and compassionate care for the person who tests positive for HIV and the complicated relationships between HIV-positive persons and the health care professionals with whom they come in contact. The obligation of professionals to treat HIV-positive persons falls largely within the realm of the principle of beneficence. In addition, the obligation of institutions and of society as a whole to treat such persons with dignity and respect is also encompassed by the principle. Again, in the body of the chapter, the principle of beneficence will be discussed, as well as the care which the person receives from individual practitioners, from institutions, and from society as a whole.

Justice

Justice is sometimes described in terms of fairness and "what is deserved." The notion of justice has been variously analyzed in different theoretical approaches. A common thread, however, common to all theories of justice, is this minimal principle: like cases should be treated alike or, equals ought to be treated equally and unequals unequally (Beauchamp and Walter 1982). The fair treatment of persons involved in HIV testing and in the outcome of such testing falls under this principle. The right to health care at any level within our society, or for any class of persons suffering from a variety of diseases, is rarely argued or implemented from the viewpoint of justice—in other words, HIV-positive patients are no different from anybody else. With its limited appreciation of justice the most that one can expect from our society for persons suffering from an HIV-positive diagnosis or from the development of AIDS is a decent minimum of care. Our ability to guarantee such a basic human minimum must be seen as an essential ethical statement, however meager, of our willingness to respect the essential humanity of persons with the HIV infection.

The principles of autonomy, non-maleficence, beneficence, and justice intertwine in their complementarity and in their conflict as one seeks to determine and develop ethical stances toward HIV testing. The challenge of the succeeding sections is to apply these principles to the issues around the need for HIV testing itself, to the type of care that should be afforded persons who test positive, to the rights of health care providers, and to the issues surrounding access to health care for those who need it because of the infection and the consequences of the infection.

THE TEST

The first step to consider in the HIV epidemic is the test used to identify those who are HIV positive. The current false-positive rate in good labs of the ELISA test is on the order of 0.0007% (Weiss 1988). Even with this unusually high specificity rate false positives will occur. As noted in the *New England Journal of Medicine*:

> Imagine testing 100,000 people, among whom the prevalence of disease is 0.01%. Of the 100,000, 10 are infected; 99,990 are not. A combination of tests that is 100% sensitive will correctly identify all 10 who are infected. If the joint false-positive rate is 0.005 %, the tests will yield false-positive results in 5 of the 99,990 people who are not infected. Thus, of the 15 positive results, 10 will come from people who are infected and 5 from people who are not infected, and the probability that infection is present in a patient with positive tests will be 67% (Meyer 1987).

The next question associated with testing is, Why test? The test has proven effective in screening blood and blood products from infection, but the test is not foolproof and infected blood may still test negative. Another rationale for testing is to discover those who are infected and treat the disease, however, an HIV infection is not treatable at this time and little is known about its progression to AIDS. Hopefully, this argument against testing will not be long lived. Current research shows that there is some advantage to early identification of HIV positivity and early treatment with AZT may slow the progression of the infection to AIDS (*New York Times*, August 21, 1989).

A third rationale is to prevent infected persons from spreading the disease. There is the hope that if people have knowledge of their HIV status they will change their behavior—a questionable assumption. Furthermore, the coercive measures that would be required, were we as a society to enforce codes to prevent the spread of the disease, would be too high a price to pay in terms of personal freedom. Another rationale for the test is for contact notification, but the confidentiality of the people involved could not be guaranteed and this, too, may be too high a price to pay. Finally there is the question of quarantining the infected population; given the incubation time and sheer numbers, this too is an impractical reason for mandatory testing (Weiss et al.). Clearly, mandatory testing is not practical nor desirable at this time.

INFORMED CONSENT

Informed consent is absolutely essential to patient autonomy. Without full understanding and knowledge of the options before them patients cannot be autonomous in their decision-making. Thus, should HIV testing be performed without the patient's consent? The HIV test is not a routine blood test and places the patient at considerable risk for negative psychosocial consequences (Howell 1988). There is no cure for the HIV infection, however, recent research suggests that early treatment with AZT may help delay the onset of AIDS in HIV-positive patients. Thus knowledge of one's HIV positivity may be beneficial. The test may be useful in reducing the risk of transmission of the disease, but given the competing interests when the patient is suspected to be at risk, full consent should be obtained prior to the drawing of the test. If the test were mandatory, the people most likely to be infected would be driven away from counseling and other services (Bayer 1988).

WHO SHOULD BE TESTED?

Who should be tested? Voluntary testing should be obtained after adequate informed consent in the following populations: active homosexuals, IV drug abusers and their sexual partners, partners of prostitutes, blood transfusion recipients, and organ recipients who have unexplained symptoms associated with ARC or AIDS. Some people are forced into routine testing, these include members of the military, federal prisoners, and blood donors. It can be argued that two of these groups imply consent because they recognize that by donating blood or joining the military the HIV will be drawn, and in the case of the military, drawn at regular intervals. Currently, prisoners are the only social group coerced into testing for HIV.

CONFIDENTIALITY

Confidentiality is an essential part of patient autonomy, as it guarantees that people's problems and secrets remain theirs. When patients are tested the greatest care must be given to protecting their confidentiality. The groups in our society that at largest risk for infection, namely the homosexual population and IV drug abusers, have been consistently ostracized and maligned. Unfortunately, the appearance of the virus in these groups almost automatically labels an HIV-positive person as a member of one of these groups. Furthermore, patients may find themselves without jobs, unable to get health and life insurance, and without friends. Since it is so easy to gain access to records, and lab data pass through so many hands, the ability to control this information becomes difficult. With automated lab testing, confidentiality of information is virtually impossible. Furthermore, some hospitals have AIDS wards and if a patient is admitted to one of these wards it is assumed that he or she must have the HIV infection.

DUTY TO WARN

Perhaps the thorniest ethical issue is the duty to warn endangered third parties. In the court decision of *Tarasoff* v. *Regents of the University of California*, a legal standard for a duty to warn endangered third parties was formulated (Dickens 1988). This will likely extend to the warning of partners of HIV-infected individuals. When is it permissible, and is it ethically responsible, to break the confidentiality of patients who refuse to tell sexual partners about their HIV positivity? Arguments against breaking the confidence include the very real concern that it would drive people in need of care and counseling further underground. There is also the question of what exposed partners would learn from the test. The issues of testing the partner are the same as those regarding testing the population at risk.

The very cogent argument for warning is to prevent further spread of the disease. There are numerous examples of required contacting of partners and forced quarantine. However, these have been associated with diseases which had a rapid course or were in some degree treatable.

All of these concerns can be classified in the scheme of patient autonomy versus the individual good of others and the overall common good. Testing can only be done if the patient is fully informed of the consequences of a positive test. Furthermore, at this stage in our understanding of the disease, the patient should receive the information that much is not known. To protect patients' autonomy and freedom to live their lives as they see fit, every effort must be made to protect their confidentiality, maybe even to the point of respecting their wish that sexual contacts not be notified of their exposure.

JUSTICE / COMMON GOOD

Justice, or social concern, has some cogent arguments. The testing of individuals would provide valuable epidemiologic data about the origin, extent, and spread of the disease. Hopefully, when individuals have knowledge of the problem, efforts will be made to stem the spread of the disease. Also, does the lack of testing condone the behavior which places a person at risk for contracting the disease? Not using the force of societal pressure as represented by the HIV test can be seen as ignoring the problem and condoning the behaviors which lead to the epidemic in the first place. However, the force of societal pressure can be brought to bear in other arenas, such as aggressive education, and drug treatment programs.

Thus it is our opinion that voluntary testing is the best option at this time. High-risk groups should be encouraged to accept the test and its consequences as a means to control the spread of the disease. Those found to be positive should be encouraged to inform their sexual partners about the problem. With such measures the spread of the disease might be curtailed. Furthermore, if the preliminary research about the efficacy of early treatment with AZT proves to be true, then taking the test would be of great benefit to the patient.

THE PROFESSIONAL RESPONSE

Another arena to be considered in testing is the response of the health care professional. Physicians and other health care providers, out of a sense of beneficence, have historically placed themselves in harm's way in order to care for the sick patient. While this has been the professional ideal, it has not always been the profession's behavior. In a thoughtful article concerning physicians behavior in the last great plague to hit London, Zuger and Mills noted that the physicians behaved poorly. Most physicians fled the city, and were soundly ridiculed and castigated for abandoning the populace at that time of great need. However, those that remained to care for the dying were also ridiculed and criticized for their ineffectiveness. Currently, there is great professional argument about the health care professional's obligation to care for the HIV-positive patient. Many physicians, in particular, feel that placing themselves at risk is uncalled for and unnecessary, and since nothing can be done there should be no moral obligation to care for the HIV-positive patient. This is a hollow argument. That there is no standard which states that health care professionals have to place themselves intentionally in harm's way has been cited by those those who propose that there is no obligation to care for the HIV patient. But the risk of contracting an HIV infection in the course of caring for a patient is infinitesimally small. Those who have converted to HIV positive in the course of treatment have done so through careless, thoughtless mistakes, or possibly deliberate suicidal intent.

Another argument that is advanced is that the health care professional has an obligation to other patients. This, too, is not a sound argument, as there is no truly indispensable health care professional. Duty to the family is another argument advanced as a reason not to care for the HIV patient. This argument has some merit. The health care professional's spouse, prior to the marriage, willingly accepted the person as a member of a profession which involves a degree of risk. However, the children of health care professionals had no choice in the matter, and should not be placed at risk of contracting a disease due to the parent's profession. However, since the risk of the parent converting to HIV positive is so small, there is virtually no chance that the children of the health care provider will be placed at risk.

Therefore, the health care provider does have a moral and ethical obligation to care for the HIV-positive patient. This obligation is based on the ethical principle of justice, as well as the traditions of the profession to care for the sick. The risk of contracting this disease appears to be small in the face of appropriate precautions. The only cogent argument against treating the HIV-infected patient is that the health care provider cannot adequately care for the HIV-positive patient due to lack of education and experience. Workers in this category should refer patients to more qualified professionals, but this will not excuse such workers from gaining education through traditional means so that they will be equipped to handle at least the initial phases of treatment and counseling. No branch of the health professions has stepped forward to claim ownership of the disease caused by HIV infection. Consequently, treatment of the HIV patient will likely remain a mishmash of various specialties.

Burn-out

The principle of beneficence obliges health care professionals to respect their own well-being in the care of the HIV-infected person. An area of particular concern is the prevention of professional burn-out. The HIV-infected patient is difficult to care for because so little is known at this time. The patients are generally young, in the prime of their lives, and at the peak of their creativity and contribution to society, matching the age and similar qualities of health professionals. Furthermore, at this time, the HIV-positive patient is viewed as being hopelessly ill, which may not be an accurate assumption. Also, at this time there is no cure for HIV infection. These factors contribute to a high burn-out rate, and health professionals should be on the watch for signs of burn-out so that it can be combated.

Ironically, since so little can be done for the disease, the HIV-positive patient represents a chance for the profession to re-establish a more personal, caring link with the patient. Many people have decried the erosion of the doctor-patient relationship and how our technology has distanced us from our patients (Time Magazine, July 31, 1989). The HIV-positive patient represents a chance to re-establish this link. Caring for the HIV-positive patient will largely be a matter of support, counseling, and monitoring for further development of the disease. If our care for these patients is to be ethical, moral, and caring, the profession must be prepared to give them the time needed to foster a true relationship. This caring link brings together in a meaningful way the fullest expression of the principles of autonomy, respect for the patient, beneficence, and justice.

Counseling

Studies show that the patients who make the poorest adjustment are those identified as positive without signs of AIDS Related Complex (ARC) or AIDS. These people must go through major lifestyle changes, and are at risk of great personal, professional, and financial loss. They will most likely go through the stages of personal grief as outlined by Kübler-Ross, Schneider, and others. Coping with these problems requires an involved and caring professional response. This disease represents a challenge to all that is good in the health care professions, and we should not shirk our responsibilities in this regard. There will be difficult questions to answer early in the treatment of HIV-infected individuals. It is known that the virus attacks the brain and causes a deterioration of mental functioning. So, early on, while the patients are still in command of their full capabilities, such questions as what measures they want taken in their treatment, and what is to be done as the condition worsens must be addressed. A caveat, this must be done in a caring, sensitive manner so as not to rob the person of the hope necessary for daily living.

RESEARCH PROBLEMS

It is important to address research ethics as they pertain to the HIV-positive patient. The nature and spread of the disease is still largely unknown because the disease is connected to sexual behavior, and human sexual behavior is a sensitive topic which is difficult to research. Intravenous drug use is another mode of transmission, and this behavior also does not lend itself easily to examination, research, and understanding. If we are to gain a full understanding of the disease and its progression, we must, of necessity, engage in meaningful, difficult research in the areas of sexuality and drug use. This means placing our own moral priorities on hold to ask these difficult questions. It also requires a commitment in dollars.

An example of the difficulty of establishing an understanding of human sexual behavior is underscored in a recent article by Weiss (1989). He describes our lack of knowledge of the extent of the sexual behavior found in the etiology of HIV infections. He exhorts us to fill "the epidemiological black hole" which is the result of our lack of understanding of the extent of "at risk" sexual behavior.

What are the ethics of a double-blind, controlled study of people who are infected? Is it ethically permissible to conduct a study is which one half of a group of ill patients, who have a high likelihood of dying, do not receive any treatment? In this setting, is informed consent possible? In order to have a truly informed consent to treatment the patient must have the mental ability to understand, and the information, including alternatives, with which to work. Furthermore, the consent must not be coerced. HIV-positive patients have the potential to fail in all regards. First, HIV infects the brain, and subtle organicity may impair the patient before any other signs of AIDS are present. Second, there is not much information about alternatives, and the bottom line is that the disease will most likely progress to death. Third, given the death sentence, any treatment which gives the potential for hope can hardly be called uncoerced.

It can be seen that HIV is giving the health care professions an opportunity to stop and reflect on their relationships to the patient, the disease, and the research. It has been humbling, especially for the medical profession, to battle this disease. In the years just prior to the emergence of HIV, the medical profession had become rather smug about its ability to fight and conquer infectious diseases. It was the widespread feeling that most of the horrible ravages of humankind had been conquered, and that what was left were occasional out-breaks of previously devastating epidemics. HIV has brought the profession back to the reality that anything can happen.

CONCLUSION

This chapter represents an effort to examine the implications of the application of the ethical principles of autonomy, non-maleficence, beneficence, and justice to selected aspects of HIV testing. Of neces-sity, this approach is wide-ranging; no claim is laid to this being an exhaustive presentation. Rather, it is a modest attempt to promote some serious reflection around the many human issues which result from HIV testing.

A recent editorial in *Ethical Currents* (November 1987), under the provocative title "Outlawing AIDS," has some excellent observations which may serve well as a conclusion to our previous discussion. The editorial aptly points out that when HIV testing is discussed in the public policy arena, the competing principles are always presented as a conflict between individual rights and public health. The article, arguing that there is a greater good involved, namely the "public good," notes:

> The public good is not synonymous with individual rights, although preserving individual rights contributes to the public good. Nor, is the public good synonymous with public health, although the public good is surely enriched by less disease. Public good speaks of the kind of society we live in and want to live in.

The editorial goes on to say that those with HIV infection should not be burdened with all of the responsibilities and risks in protecting human health, while the uninfected receive all the benefits. Similarly, the uninfected should not run all the risks of caring for the infected, while they in turn remain unprotected.

It would seem that the ethical principles which address the ethi-cal issues surrounding HIV testing call for a balancing of the rights of all involved. The presence of HIV-infected persons in our society is a challenge to our capacity to engage in careful ethical analysis of the basic values and issues involved. Ambiguity and uncertainty are to be expected in dealing with the ethical issues surrounding HIV testing, and the human predicaments which result from it. It seems that we are called in this disease, as in other fatal diseases, to create a true community of care in which the human dignity of all persons involved is assured. Ethical reflection on the part of all involved, in whatever aspect of HIV testing, should promote within such persons a keener appreciation of their own humanity.

Ethical principles and ethical reflection of themselves do not necessarily promote a more humane society. One must concur with the observation of Beauchamp and Childress (1989) that for every moral principle and rule there is a corresponding virtue, that is a corresponding trait or disposition to act. They suggest that from autonomy flows respectfulness, that from beneficence flows benevolence, that from justice comes fairness. Fidelity and faithfulness, veracity and truthfulness, and the other desirable virtues which are needed to deal with the human crisis surrounding HIV infection can be promoted by honest, ethical reflection.

Treating and caring for people with the HIV infection, and the subsequent development of AIDS, provides the healthcare profession with the opportunity to reflect on its values and its relationship to the patient. Zuger (1987), commenting on the experience of residents caring for the AIDS patient writes:

> ... their ethical training has been unparalleled—practical, comprehensive and complete beyond that received by any physicians today or in recent memory.

A Presidential Commission (1983) which the studied ethical problems surrounding access to health care reminds us:

> the depth of society's concern about health care can be seen as a measure of its solidarity in the face of suffering and death. As society's commitment to health care reflects some of its most basic attitudes about what it means to be a member of the human community.

Surely this has special meaning when applied to the care of persons with the HIV infection.

Barrett (1989), a recent commentator on the human dimensions of counseling persons with the HIV infection, notes that the present time constitutes the "easy days of the AIDS virus." He also notes:

> the depth of society's concern about health care can be seen as a measure of its solidarity in the face of suffering and death. As society's

commitment to health care reflects some of its most basic attitudes about what it means to be a member of the human community.

Barrett concludes:

those facing AIDS are our brothers and sisters, our sons and daughters, our mothers and fathers. Reaching out to them with love and commitment can become a significant professional and humanitarian activity.

REFERENCES

Barrett, R.L. 1989. Counseling gay men with AIDS: human dimension. *J. Counseling Dev.* 67, 10:573–575.

Bayer, R. 1988. Screening and AIDS: the limits of coercive intervention *Ann. N.Y. Acad. Sci.* 530:159–62.

Beauchamp, T.L. and L. Walters. 1982. *Contemporary Issues in Bioethics,* 2nd ed. Belmont, CA: Wadsworth.

Beauchamp, T.L. and J.F. Childress. 1989. *Principles of Biomedical Ethics,* 3rd Ed. New York: Oxford University Press.

Dickens, B.M. Legal limits of AIDS confidentiality. *J.A.M.A.* 259, 23: 3449–3451.

Doctors and patients. *Time,* July 31, 1989.

Dyer, A.L. 1988. AIDS, ethics and psychiatry. *Psychiatric Ann.* 18, 10:577–581.

Frankena, W.K. 1973. *Ethics,* 2nd Ed. Englewood Cliffs, NJ: Prentice Hall.

Howell, J. 1988. What is the difference between an HIV and a CBC? *Hastings Center Rep.* (August/September):18–20.

Meyer, K.B. and S.G. Pauker. 1987. *Screening for HIV: can we afford the false positive rate? N. Eng. J. Med.* 317, 4 (July 23):238–241.

New York Times, August 21, 1989; Outlawing AIDS. Ethical Currents. Orange, CA: Center for Bioethics, St. Joseph's Health System 13:1–8.

President's Commission for the Study of Ethical Problems in Medicine and Biomedical and Behavioral Research. Securing Access to Health Care 1. Washington, DC: U.S. Government Printing Office.

Weiss, R. and S.O. Thier. 1988. HIV testing is the answer—what's the question? *N. Eng. J. Med.* 319, 15 (October 13):1010–1012.

Zuger, A. 1987. AIDS on the ward: a residency in medical ethics. *Hasting Center Rep.* (June):16–20.

Zuger, A. and S.H. Miles. 1987. Physician, AIDS and occupational risk: historical tradition and ethical obligations. *J.A.M.A.* 258, 14 (October 9): 1924–1928.

6

From Shock to Re-Engagement: Learning the Diagnosis

Beverly A. Hall, RN, PhD, FAAN, and Janet D. Allan, RN, PhD

This chapter reports on how a person deals with learning that he is seropositive for the human immunodeficiency virus (HIV). Interviews that lasted from 4 to 8 hours were conducted with 11 gay men in the asymptomatic stage (stage II) of HIV disease. These informants were confronting the task of living with the diagnosis of seropositivity for the human immunodeficiency virus, a condition that scientists have said is 100% fatal over an 8-year period (Institute of Medicine, National Academy of Science, 1988).

The data on which this chapter is based were sifted from a larger data collection that was done to document help-seeking patterns among this population (Allan and Hall 1989). Much of this information appeared as serendipitous and unexpected findings. We realized halfway through the process that these men were trying to talk about something more basic than their help-seeking. They were talking about how to reclaim life itself, about the process of re-engagement in life after receiving a potentially terminal diagnosis.

Although data were cross-sectional, both recall data and analysis of data by time-since-testing-seropositive suggest a rather consistent pattern of response including initial shock followed by anger, uncertainty, anxiety, then finally a change of outlook, taking contol of one's life, redefining reality and re-engagement with life. Informants reported a wide range of behavioral and emotional responses to finding out that they were seropositive, which included feeling depressed, fearful, angry at God and the world; engaging in excessive drinking; and taking drugs. Most believed their lives were over.

Dealing with the the fact of seropositivity was an individual and lonely process for many of these informants because the health care system seemed to have no answers, only bad news. One 25-year-old man, told that he was seropositive for HIV disease, said:

Emotionally, I did the usual first thing. I broke down and cried. I started trying to work it through. Went into a depression. Started to read a little, but it was so depressing. I also had some feelings of anger. Not helpful anger. I did not go to a support group, because I was afraid the people would be more concerned with dying than living.

Another said:

I did a lot of drinking and drugs. I was real upset and I got plastered a lot. I thought, what is the use? I am going to die anyway. I also did drugs to forget about it. I was just very angry at the world and at God for doing this to me.

Almost all the persons we interviewed went through a self-destructive and angry period while they were dealing with the initial impact of their diagnosis. Another man, aged 23, who had learned about his positive test only a month before the interview, said:

I worked in gay bars off and on for three years as a bartender. I got sick of it and I never would drink myself. I lost tips because I would'nt let people buy me a drink. Here I am now, drinking and doing cocaine and AIDS positive. My job is killing me. I am pushing drugs to pay for school. What a mess. I am sick, ugly, dirty. When the call came, I said, 'goodbye.' I am the plague. In the gay life everything is appearance. If I get K.S., I'll shoot myself.

Another said:

With me, the raw fear lasted a month. A support group that I went to scared the hell out of me. It was a lot of non-positive-type older AIDS people. All they talked about was dying. That scared the hell out of me. When I left that night, all that I could think of was, I'm dead. Couple of months I would be dead.

Although grief and death are as much cultural processes as biosocial processes, the shock a person experiences upon receiving a terminal diagnosis has received very little attention. The very subject of death is regarded as painful in Western society, even among health professionals and academics. In another study we explored the literature about this phase in an article, "Between Diagnosis and Death: The Case for Studying Grief Before Death" (1988). We found that the little research that had been done concerned people who were in the physiological stages of dying, and on grief responses of parents, widows and children. We did not find any systematic studies on the shock of receiving a terminal diagnosis except that done on uncertainty after receiving a cancer diagnosis.

The literature on the response to terminal diagnosis consists largely of personal accounts written by physicians, nurses, and articulate patients and family members (Cousins 1979, 1983; Siegal 1988; Mullan 1983). Because of early detection of disease, people are living much longer with a view of their impending death, and they are being medicalized and segregated from the healthy. One account by a young physician who discovered that he had cancer was typical. It dealt with the limbo state that occurred after his diagnosis (Mullan 1983). He described how different he felt from those around him, his complete subservience to the medical system, his anger at his caretakers and his body, and the complete frustration he experienced regarding how to pick up his life again and who to tell.

Something that is seldom written about in the professional literature is the phase of resuming one's life following a terminal diagnosis. This stage involves the rediscovery of hope. If patients can learn to cope by gaining self-control and a positive attitude toward the outcome, they describe this period as one of the happiest in their lives. They begin to incorporate their experiences into a renewed philosophy of life. They look for hope and health. This period is characterized by attention to self-fulfillment, opportunities for personal growth and stability, emotional maturity, self-determination, personal satisfaction, enthusiasm, and happiness.

At the outset, most informants found out from a physician that they were seropositive. Many had suspected that they were infected, but most expressed surprise when they actually were told. The usual reason for having the test was a suggestion by the doctor to whom they went with a minor complaint. Two were tested because their partners had tested positive. The first reaction on hearing the news was one of shock that lasted from 2 to 6 weeks. Most thought that they would be dead within a very short time, that their lives were finished. One person said:

> I just want to know that there was one other person in the world who had my diagnosis, who lived. Just one other person, and knowing that would give me hope that I might make it into that ten percent that overcome this.

Later he said that it was that struggle to regain health that not only kept him alive, but also moved him into the realm of the truly living. He understood what was important to him. More emphasis was put on positive relationships and life that was productive and useful.

For those who are going to fight to attain health, their task at this point is one that leads them into strong emotions, a great deal of anger, fear, rejection of the diagnosis, and rejection of their caretakers. Then something usually happens that sets the person in a more positive direction.

One informant said:

> It's funny because things seem so simple now. I went through a lot— trauma, turmoil. I look back now and feel that I wasted a lot of my time and energy in being upset. The most important thing I did was to change my attitude and outlook. Don't accept a death sentence. Don't feel like you are a victim. You are AIDS positive, but you can live with it.

This period of turmoil, however, was common to almost all the men in the study. Whether it is a necessary part of the process, we cannot judge. What we do suspect is that those who "go gentle into that good night" are not the survivors. Those are the ones who will die. Other observers, such as Cousins (1979, 1983) and Siegel (1986) have described the same process.

One of our informants who has lived 4 years in an asymptomatic state experienced more depression than anger in the beginning:

> I had a 3-month period in which I would get up in the morning, smoke pot, sit and look out the window and find myself unable to get up and perform any one of a hundred enjoyable tasks that involved working on things near and dear to me. It just came to me all of a sudden that all it takes is just you dealing with the changes. There is the grim reality out there that if you get sick, you are going to die. That is the grim reality of being on earth. If I get sick, I will deal with it then. I would never think that I would have dealt with all this as nobly as I am dealing with it.

Thus the first stage of shock is characterized by anger, anxiety or depression, a reliance drugs or alcohol, and a sort of giving up. All but three of the ten men that we interviewed described this process. One man said that he never lost hope. He was self-described optimist, who credited his mental and spiritual makeup as well as the fact that he has inherited genes of longevity from his family as the reasons for his happiness. He also said:

> It did not bother me at all because I expected it. I've been positive for over 2 years and have felt very healthy the whole time. I don't think I'll get AIDS.

The other two men were absorbed in the care of their companions who were ill with AIDS, and declared that they had not yet dealt with their own problems. One of the men in this latter group died after his interview, January 23, 1989, 3 months after his companion died. He died of his very first opportunistic infection *Pneumocystis carinii* pneumonia. His lack of will to live after his partner's death was painfully clear to us during the last 3 months of his life. The investigators spent a great deal of time with him talking about his feelings and what he wanted to do with the rest of his life. His future was expressed in the vaguest terms possible. He pushed other people away from him. He was very passive in his approach to getting help. He did not want to get close to people. He spent most of his awake time watching television. On the last day of his life, we came to the hospital after taking his dog and his cat to new homes, because he knew that he could no longer care for them, and they had been sadly neglected. When we came into his room he asked about the animals, then he asked to be able to hold our hands, and then he died about 30 minutes later, totally unexpectedly, as he had been scheduled to go home the next day. His short relationship with the companion who had died represented all the happiness he had ever had in his rather lonely life. He made it clear that his hope resided in moving to a future where he felt he could be rejoined with his partner. His life on earth was quite sorrowful and lonely, as in some ways was his death. We felt that once his companion, the dog, and the cat had been accounted for, he regarded his obligations as finished and had no reason to go on. He was the one man we interviewed in our study of help-seeking who was not using any personal or self-care strategies to improve his health. His life was hopeless in the true sense of the definition by Stuart and Sundeen (1987), who define hopelessness as an individual's belief that neither he nor anyone else can do anything to aid him.

For those who experienced definite periods of shock and anger, some form of coping was not far behind. These men had to find a way to get some sort of control over their lives and their diagnosis.

It was not totally clear what factors influenced this change. The data suggested that talking to friends and family, receiving some ititial information from the physician, and personal soul searching all contributed to informants beginning to alter their attitudes. The pathway from initial shock to resolution was not linear: regression to the stage of fear, anxiety, and signs of initial crisis usually followed the development of perceived or actual symptoms that suggested changes in health status, such as a sore throat or a skin rash.

One person who had been diagnosed only 2 months before, and was going through a self-destructive period at the time of the interview, began to get involved in alternative therapy, primarily therapeutic touch. As a result, his anxiety has diminished and he is looking forward to a better year in school. He said:

Once I got into being more positive, things started falling into place. I am not scared anymore. I can handle this situation.

Another man, when asked what advice he would give to others in his situation, said:

Don't take your fears too seriously, because you can make your worst dreams come true.

This sentiment was also voiced by others.

Two of the men who live together believe that they are never going to die of AIDS. They are busy, happier than they have ever been before, volunteering at AIDS Services Organization, helping others, getting involved politically in the fight to find more resources for research and treatment of AIDS. I think that the belief that they are not going to die of AIDS is an attempt to normalize their lives so that they can extract some enjoyment from it. They do not want to be "AIDS victims." One of them said:

We have good days and bad days. That is no reason to give up. We are going to die of the same thing that anyone dies of. We are not going to die of AIDS.

All the survivors in this study, as a part of the resolution, began to see a future again and to set priorities. They begin to have needed dental work done, to return to useful occupations, to re-establish relationships with friends and lovers, to re-engage with family members, and in the case of two men, to pursue degrees at the university. One of the latter informants told us that he still has concerns about returning to school:

I still sometimes have concerns, that the things I want to do cost money, such as graduate school, in terms of whether or not that's feasible, like throwing good money after bad, should something happen that I would become ill tomorrow or 2 weeks after getting my graduate degree. The other thing is the fact that I do get something out of going to school. It's not just for a career, but for the emotions.

DISCUSSION

The expressions of hope and the process of hope described in this study of 11 men illustrate a phenomenon which this chapter attempts to document by telling the story of how they achieved hope and what it did for their lives. Perhaps our culturally learned fears of dying do not allow people in this society to prepare for death, or to fully understand the meaning of their lives until they are hit with the possibility that their lives might end soon. When these men had recovered from their initial shock, they reported a renewed appetite for life and a feeling that life was better, more settled than it had been before the diagnosis.

The persons that we interviewed were young, in good health, and had a lot going on in their lives. They had many people, friends, therapists and others who showed an outpouring of caring that helped them in their quest to take control of their lives. Still, they had to struggle for months in depression, anger, loneliness, grief and pain. It was many months before they could regain their sense of humanness, establish control over their lives and re-engage in normal activities.

Persons who work with clients along the HIV trajectory need to be able to support their efforts to change their outlook. Many studies have connected hope and optimism with longevity (Vaux 1981, Stoner and Keampfer 1985, Miller 1989). Whether longevity is the issue or not, persons who test positive usually have many more years to live, and it makes no sense to waste these years coping with impending disease or suffering from depression. It is not giving people a false sense of reality to tell them that they can have a productive and happy future. On the contrary, when we do not relate to them in a future-oriented way, and join them in the false belief that their lives are finished, we are promoting a sense of doom that has no basis in reality. Although the number of years that these men live may be shorter than it would have been had they not contracted HIV, the quality of the remaining years, we are convinced, will be greater.

Clearly death is not the enemy. Kübler-Ross (1975) said that the dying fear two things, loss of hope and abandonment. We are all going to die. The enemy is losing hope, being given up on, being cast anchorless into an unknown future by people who have already labeled one as dead.

The men in the study also figured out that death and life were not matters that were confined to being seropositive. A persistent message was that having a potentially terminal diagnosis helped them realize that everyone is going to die, and nobody really knows when. The key is to focus on living, and not to worry about the form one's death would take. One informant said:

> I finally realized that (AIDS) was just one possible way of meeting your death. So I repeated over and over to myself, "shot by an irate Iranian, crashing in an airplane, being killed in a car wreck, being shot at random by a pasing bullet or something like that," and started just statistic-counting, and came to the honest-to-God realization that my chances of

being killed in a car wreck or being shot while walking down Sixth Street, statistically, was greater than dying of AIDS in the next 5 years. That little tidbit of information was all I needed to push it a little bit further out of my reality. In this way I learned to manage my destiny, circumstances, and situations. I think that is the whole clue to survival of being seropositive.

Almost uniformly, our informants said, "When I die, I will die. I will handle that. Right now, I am going to live, I stay away from people who are not positive in their attitudes and not into living. I want to concentrate on living." And the fact is, that is exactly what most are trying earnestly to do.

The following diagram summarizes the process following the diagnosis of HIV seropositivity from initial shock to final re-engagement (Figure 1). Between the beginning and the end are several stages that

SHOCK

↓

ANGER, FEAR, ANXIETY, DEPRESSION

↓

INTERVENTION
- Services
- Friend
- Healing Techniques
- Experiencing/Caring

↓

CHANGE OF OUTLOOK

↓

TAKING CONTROL

↓

REDEFINING REALITY

↓

RE-ENGAGEMENT

Figure 1.
The process following HIV diagnosis.

involve changing one's outlook, taking control of one's life, and redefining reality. These stages need further investigation and more explication.

REFERENCES

Allan, J.D. and B.A. Hall. 1989. Help-seeking actions of seropositive gay men: An ethnographic study. Presented at the Conference on Men's Health: Alliance of Men in Nursing. San Francisco, CA.

Allan, J.D. and B.A. Hall. 1988. Between diagnosis and death: The case for studying grief before death. *Arch. Psychiatric Nursing 2*, 1:191–199.

Cousins, N. 1979. *Anatomy of an Illness As Perceived by the Patient.* New York: W.W. Norton.

Cousins, N. 1983. *The Healing Heart.* New York: Avon.

Institute on Medicine and National Academy of Sciences. 1988. *Confronting AIDS: Update 1988.* Washington DC: National Academy Press.

Kübler-Ross, E. 1975. *Death: The Final Stage of Growth.* Englewood Cliffs, NJ: Prentice-Hall.

Miller, J.F. 1989. Hope-inspiring strategies of the critically ill. *Applied Nursing Res. 2*:23–29.

Mullan, F. 1983. *Vital Signs.* New York: Dell.

Siegal, B.H. 1988. *Love, Medicine and Miracles.* New York: Harper & Row.

Stoner, M. and S.H. Keampfer. 1985. Recalled life expectancy information, phase of illness and hope in cancer patients. *Res. Nursing Health. 8*: 269–274.

Stuart, G.W. and S.J. Sundeen. 1987. *Principles and Practices of Psychiatric Nursing,* 3rd ed. St. Louis: C.V. Mosby.

Vaux, K.L. 1981. *Will to Live, Will to Die.* Minneapolis, MN: Augsburg Publishing House.

7

Pre-Test and Post-Test Counseling

Kathleen M. Nokes, PhD, RN

Each client arrives at the decision to participate in HIV testing by a different path. Some may come out of choice or curiosity; others out of fear or mandate. Although the clients come by different paths, there are identified commonalities. Many clients facing the possibility of a life-threatening illness begin to re-examine their own mortality. Thus, the health care provider in the counseling session will need a variety of skills to assist the client to manage this difficult decision and the ensuing results. Knowledge of HIV pathophysiology and treatment, patience, flexibility, and naturally, the willingness to listen, are just a few of the characteristics required in an HIV counselor.

PRE-TEST COUNSELING FOR HIV TESTING

Competent Individuals

In this situation, a competent person is anyone, regardless of age, who is mature enough to give informed consent for HIV testing. State laws vary and have an impact on age requirements and should be consulted. For example in New York State any person, regardless of age, can consent to HIV testing if he or she is able to understand the necessary information and give informed consent. Circumstances related to minors and mentally incompetent persons are unique and will be addressed in a separate section of this chapter.

The Setting

The interview should take place in a setting that offers privacy for the client. If the client has symptoms requiring hospitalization, he or she still needs to be well enough to understand the necessary informa-

Special thanks to Dorothy E. Hickey, MA, RNC for her editorial assistance.

tion. Although these requirements may seem basic, they are some-what difficult to achieve in a four-bedded hospital room when the client has, say, a 103° F temperature and is being treated for bacterial endocarditis. Because of the implications of this disease for significant others, the client should initially be approached when he or she is alone.

Differences Related to Initiation of HIV Testing

The health care provider's approach will differ according to whether the idea for HIV testing has been initiated by the provider or by the client. If during the health history interview, the provider learns that the client has participated in high-risk behaviors such as IV drug use, HIV infection should be ruled out in order to make a differential diagnosis. The provider will need to introduce the idea of HIV testing with the client. The client, despite the tremendous media exposure on this problem, may still be denying that there is any risk of infection. The provider's suggestion that the client consent to HIV testing may then invoke surprise, and perhaps anger. The provider then needs to clearly explain to the client that there are direct benefits to knowing one's HIV status. The provider can explain that through this knowl-edge, a treatment plan can be developed which will focus on effective interventions. A more comprehensive workup is no longer necessary and other diagnostic tests may be avoided. For example, in an IV drug-using client with anemia, a bone marrow aspiration would not be necessary if it was known that he was HIV positive. The etiology of the anemia would have been identified as related to HIV infection.

If the client has not previously considered himself or herself at risk for HIV infection, it is important to give the person enough time to consider the decision about HIV testing. By not forcing a client to decide precipitously, it may be more likely that he will agree to testing and perhaps be more prepared to deal with positive results as well. The time to consider the decision can vary from a few minutes to a day depending upon the specific circumstances. To achieve the long-term goals of building trust and promoting responsible behavior, this less-ening of time pressure is crucial.

Initiating the Counseling Session

Even when the clients have initiated contact with the health care pro-vider, the interview should begin with an open-ended question such as, "What brings you here today?" The initial response may yield a wealth of information about the client's knowledge, clarity about testing, and motivation. Responses may range from "to be tested for the AIDS virus" to "because my parole officer sent me," or "my husband is being treated here for AIDS and he said that I should come." From the diversity of these answers, it is readily apparent that the interview can take a number of different directions. It may be helpful to use an assessment form such as the one outlined in this chapter to ensure that all the necessary data are communicated and that the interview doesn't evolve tangentially, resulting in the neglect of essential components. It is not unusual for a counselor to interview from six to eight clients per day and an assessment form can be useful to note information during the interview and then to write up the interaction more formally in the client's chart.

Sharing Information

Once the client is clear about the purpose of the interaction, a dialogue can begin. The health care provider must ensure that the client understands that the test reveals whether HIV antibodies are present. At the same time, it is important to point out that current evidence indicates that HIV antibodies in clients over 15 months of age means presence of the virus and probably development of AIDS at some undetermined point in the future.

     The client needs to know that a positive test alone gives little indication of time of infection because the incubation period is anywhere from 5 to 10 years. This point needs reinforcement especially if the test is positive and the client is blaming a sexual partner of 10 months. That partner can indeed be the person who transmitted the virus in an HIV-positive person without symptoms, but if symptoms are present a recent partner is an unlikely source of infection. Some people, especially women who don't perceive themselves as engaging in any risk behaviors, but who have been sexually active with men who used IV drugs, may want to identify the person who may have transmitted the virus to them. In the pretesting situation, it needs to be clarified that transmission could have occurred at any point during the preceding 5 to 10 years.

     Describing the continuum of HIV infection to an anxious client can be a challenge. While clients need to be able to differentiate between HIV infection and AIDS, they cannot be led to believe that they are two different problems. Some clients will remark, "I have the virus, but I don't have AIDS, so that's not so bad." Clients need to know that while there are differences in terms of treatment and prognosis, no one has yet to develop AIDS without first having had the HIV virus. Drawing simple pictures of a straight line and breaking it

into incubation period, symptoms, and AIDS, and giving approxi-
mate lengths of time, helps to clarify the continuum in the client's
mind. Self-help measures that can be taken at various points along the
HIV continuum should be emphasized, while giving an explanation
of the disease process.

The disease and its transmission, as well as most discussions of
HIV infection, are fraught with issues of confidentiality and discrimination. If a medical chart is being created, the client should understand who will have access to the document. At anonymous testing
sites, there is often minimal documentation; clients who are anxious
about confidentiality issues might be more comfortable if referred to
one of those settings. Concerns about confidentiality should be introduced by the interviewer. The client can then be encouraged to explore
whether to share with anyone else that she or he is being tested for the
HIV infection. When printed patient-teaching material is distributed,
the client should be alerted to the possibility that others might perceive possession of this information as suspicious and equate it with
someone having had the disease. In some states HIV testing is free,
but even when a client has health insurance, she or he should be
counseled carefully about whether to submit a claim to the insurance
company for reimbursement for the visit. Test results can only be
given to the person consenting to the test and these results will only
be given in person. Although it can be confusing, clients should be
advised that information about significant others will not be shared
without that person's expressed consent. Any exceptions should be
discussed with the client before testing. Attention to these issues will
build the client's trust in the counselor.

A client requesting HIV testing should be assessed for HIV-
related symptoms. If the providers in the facility doing the testing will
also be giving subsequent care, it is helpful to determine a baseline
blood pressure, pulse, respirations, temperature, and weight. There
is often a 3-week delay between testing and the post-testing interview. If the test results are positive, physical changes can occur during
that period.

The assessment tool (Figure 1) addresses common health care
problems associated with HIV infection. While the purpose of HIV
counseling is certainly not to give primary care, this interaction may
be the first time that a client has seen anyone associated with health
care in a number of years. Assessing for HIV-related symptoms has a
number of benefits. First, it facilitates identification of problems that
need immediate intervention. For example, although one client did
not seem in any unusual distress, his temperature was 105° F. After
blood was drawn for HIV, he was sent to the emergency room via

Figure 1.
HIV Assessment Tool

Name _____ Date _____ Age ____
Support system _____ Risk behavior_____
Prior HIV testing: Yes __ No __ When?____ Where? _____
Children: Yes ____ Ages _____ Tested? ____
Drug treatment program _____

Symptoms Associated with HIV Infection

                                                                    Yes   No
Fatigue
Rapid weight loss
Diarrhea
Shortness of breath
Cough
Night sweats, chills
Fever
Swollen lymph nodes: Cervical __ Axillary __ Groin __
Thrush
Skin rash
Unusual bleeding
   (if female, investigate menses)
Dizziness
Headache
Peripheral neuropathy
Eye problems

Contacts

Sexual partner: Male ____ Female ____ Tested: Yes ____ No ____

Counseled

Safer sex ___ Drug use paraphernalia ___ ADL interventions ___

Printed material given:

ambulance and was sick enough to be admitted to the intensive care unit. In other cases, clients who were unaware that the white patches on their tongues were caused by a fungus, attempted to remove them with a toothbrush, thereby worsening a problem that can be properly treated with medication. The counselor needs to know when to refer clients with health care problems to other providers.

Second, while the counselor is assessing possible HIV symptoms, the client becomes aware of the problems that relate to HIV infection. Knowledge of what constitutes HIV-related symptoms can assist the person to avoid seeking care from other health care providers who may not be considering HIV infection in their diagnostic workup. For example, a client with a history of IV drug use went to a podiatrist for foot pain. The podiatrist, focusing on the presenting symptom, prescribed Tylenol with codeine. However, the underlying problem was peripheral neuropathy associated with HIV infection.

Third, assessing HIV-related symptoms helps both counselor and client anticipate the probable results of the HIV test. This is not to say that clients who manifest no symptoms should be falsely reassured that they will probably test negative. It is to say that if a client has lymphadenopathy and thrush with a recent history of IV drug use, he should be warned that the outcome of the test will probably indicate an HIV infection.

During the pre-test counseling session, the interviewer should gather information that may be helpful during the post-test session. It can be useful to determine what the client perceives will be the test results. It is particularly meaningful to explore how the client anticipates he or she will respond if the test is positive. Some clients may be at risk for suicide attempts during the period immediately after learning their test results. A client may be able to express or somehow indicate this during the pre-test period.

Clients should be encouraged to consider whether they want a support system available after the post-test visit so that they can plan to ask someone to accompany them to the session. The interviewer should not assume, however, that the significant other has been told about the purpose of the visit. For example, a woman who had had one extramarital affair which she thought had exposed her to HIV infection was accompanied to the clinic by her husband and child, but she never told them the purpose of the visit. The client should be asked if the significant other should be present when the results are shared and, if so, every effort should be made to provide for this.

During the pre-test session, the client should be advised that contacts must be notified if the client is HIV positive. According to New York Sate law, for example, the client is encouraged to tell contacts but he or she refuses to share this information, the client is made aware that either the physician or the public health officer will notify contacts. This disclosure needs to be clarified before the client consents to HIV testing. It is imperative that interviewers are familiar with the state laws which will impact on their HIV-related practice.

During the pre-test counseling session, the client should be educated about safer sex practices. Up-to-date information about decreasing HIV transmission through safer sexual practices should be conveyed to the client. It is helpful to have samples of condoms, dental dams, and contraceptive foams and creams available. In order to apply a basic principle of learning, the clients should receive verbal instruction reinforced by written material and illustrations. The counselor's preconceptions about the client's behavior should not limit the information to be provided. By creating an atmosphere in which the client feels free to share information, specific points can be emphasized. Examples include use of a water-soluble lubricant in addition to condoms during anal sex and special care to be used during oral sex if the sexual partner is known to be HIV positive. Explicit words and descriptions should be used, but not to the point that the client is too embarrassed to identify with that behavior.

If the client continues to use illegal drugs, counseling should include information about the possible consequences of that behavior. IV drug users need to know not only how to clean syringes and other drug-related paraphernalia; knowing the incidence of HIV infection in their community can help clients to understand the risks of contracting the HIV infection. For example, if in a particular community the incidence of HIV infection is 80% in IV drug users, the person needs to know that there are 8 chances in 10 of being infected if he or she continues to share drug equipment. An offer should be made to assist the client to enter into a drug treatment program. Phone calls can be made and letters written by the counselor rather than just giving the client the name and address of an agency. In a large city like New York, it is incredibly difficult to enter into a drug treatment program, and clients often must have advocates to help them through the maze. A central agency that is knowledgeable about available treatment programs and vacancies such as ADAPT (a New York City-based referral service) can be an excellent resource. The role of the HIV counselor is one of facilitator, not intercessor, with respect to the client's drug use. The client must understand clearly that continued use of drugs accelerates the disease process. It is also important to recognize the diversity among IV drug users and to treat each person as an individual, taking into consideration the kind, frequency, and amount of the drug being used.

The pre-test session takes from 30 to 45 minutes. Printed information about HIV infection developed by different voluntary and public sources is given during this session to reinforce specific points. By being sensitive to verbal and nonverbal clues from the client, the counselor can encourage questions.

Agencies usually require written consent and these forms often address similar concerns to those which have been discussed in the interview. The client is encouraged to read the informed consent form carefully and sign only after all questions have been satisfactorily answered. It is advisable to point out that if the test results are negative, periodic re-testing—usually every 3 months—is indicated for at least 9 months after the identified risk behavior. The client is cautioned that a negative result, while hopeful, is not conclusive. It is often helpful to show the client any forms that are being used and to point out the number which identifies the blood sample. This can assist in reassuring the client that the actual testing is individual, personal, and anonymous.

SPECIAL CASES

Women of Childbearing Age

Women in childbearing years will require a more in-depth assessment in certain areas. The woman needs to understand that if she is seropositive, being pregnant will have an impact on both herself and the unborn child. Current literature on HIV infection and pregnancy indicates that the stress of pregnancy may accelerate the HIV disease process. The possibility of the child being born HIV positive ranges from 20% to 50% and it is as yet unclear how many of those children will remain HIV positive after 15 to 18 months of age (Reference Manual, 1988, p. 13). The routine waiting period of 2 to 3 weeks between testing and learning the results will need to be shortened if the woman is considering an abortion. If termination of pregnancy is not an option, then the woman will require special counseling should her test results be positive.

Minors

If the minor is mature enough to understand the information, he or she should be treated as an adult in the HIV counseling session. The situation is more complex in younger children. If the child is under 5 years of age, the parent or legal guardian needs to give consent for the child. If the child is in foster care, it is essential to ensure that the legal guardian is the one who is actually giving the consent for HIV testing. There are a number of legal and economic considerations related to the child's HIV status. It is better to proceed cautiously than to find oneself in the situation of needing to answer the question, "who authorized the testing of this HIV-positive infant?" The rights of the natural parents, the foster parents, the foster care agency, and most importantly, of the child, need to be weighed carefully.

Mentally Retarded Clients

State laws will affect who will give consent for HIV testing for mentally retarded clients. If those clients can understand the information, they can consent. If their mental age precludes understanding, then specific laws and policies should be consulted on how to proceed. HIV testing would not be considered an emergency procedure, so rules established for consent in elective situations is applicable.

Prisoners

Local, state, and federal laws also have an impact on prisoners and HIV testing. In some situations, prisoners may not be allowed to refuse testing but they still should be counseled about HIV infection. Confidentiality is particularly sensitive when working with prisoners, since access to patient data is so readily accessible and authority figures in the environment can be intimidating.

POST-TEST COUNSELING

The counselor should review the test results before meeting with the client. It is not unusual to feel a sense of relief at receiving a client's negative results. Positive results, on the other hand, often bring a sense of dread—of not wanting to tell the client, of sadness for the person, and concern about how he will react. By working through these feelings before meeting with the client, the counselor can be more sensitive in responding to the client's reaction.

To prepare for the meeting with the client, the counselor reviews the records from the pre-test session, which will help in recalling what the client's anticipated response to the results may be. It is always helpful to provide continuity by having the person who did the pre-test counseling also reveal the test results. If the client wants a significant other to be part of the post-test session, both should be invited into the private area.

The client is probably experiencing some anxiety about what the counselor is about to say. The waiting period between testing and hearing the test results is often a time of reflection on one's life and making resolutions. Once everyone has settled into the interview, the results should be shared with the client. Be very sensitive to the client's initial response. If it seems helpful, touch the client gently. Tissues should be readily available. Give the client time to process the information.

When the Test Results are Negative

It is important not to abbreviate the post-test session for a client with negative HIV test results. After the joy has been shared, the interview needs to refocus on why testing was perceived as necessary. Prevention measures need to be strongly reinforced. If the risk behavior was within the last 6 months, the person should return for periodic HIV testing every 3 months until the window period, the time between infection and a change in test results, has safely passed. Current thinking is that the window period can range from 6 weeks to a year. A follow-up appointment for retesting should be made during this post-test visit.

There are at least two options if a client who presented with symptoms is HIV negative. One is that the test results reflect a false negative and this client should be advised to have retesting for HIV. Another option is that the client has a different health care problem such as diabetes or cancer. Referrals need to be made to primary health care providers so that a more complete workup can be done.

Clients often appreciate receiving a copy of the test results. It serves to reassure them that a mistake has not been made. The client can also share these results with appropriate others. If a copy is made available, remind the client to reveal the information very cautiously because it may be difficult to predict the reaction of others. The person may become curious about the initial motivation for HIV testing and the client may not want to reveal this information.

When the Test Results are Positive

Clients often react to positive test results as if they have just received a death sentence. If there is an unusually long silence after hearing the results, it may be helpful to ask the client what is being experienced. Let the client react at his or her own pace, but don't let the client precipitously terminate the interview. If the person stands up and says, "Well, that's it," ask him to sit down again. The client may be experiencing an emotional roller coaster ride and the counselor should try to maintain contact. Once the initial period of the post-test interview is over and the client knows his HIV status, additional information needs to be conveyed. Maintain a hopeful, yet realistic attitude. Don't promise cures, but also reinforce that the prognosis associated with HIV infection has improved greatly as new treatment options have been made available.

Assess the client's readiness to hear new information. At least two factors may intervene: anxiety and HIV-related dementia. The latter may be subtle but, if present, will interfere with conceptual abilities. Once the client has processed the information about antibody status, there may be questions. Let the client direct this part of the session by indicating what he needs to know.

There is also certain information that the counselor must convey. The question of transmitting the virus to significant others needs to be reintroduced. Now, this person needs to be told that he or she also needs to be tested for HIV infection. This can be quite complex. The man may not have told his wife that he is bisexual. The woman may not have told her husband that she uses drugs. The man may not have told his wife that he has had extramarital affairs. The HIV positive person is being faced not only with his or her HIV status but also with the possibility that the responsibility for spreading the virus rests with him or her. The counselor needs to be gentle and yet firm. Help the client process how the information about HIV infection will be shared. Offer assistance in speaking with the significant other. Suggest that the significant other can also be seen by the counselor for testing but assure the client that confidentiality will be maintained.

Some state laws require notification of significant others if the client refuses to share the information. The client should be reminded of this and alerted that the significant other will be contacted. Alerting contacts activates a number of possible responses. A violent reaction can precipitate murder or suicide; a rejecting response can result in breakup of the family and loss of a home and access to children; while an accepting reaction can be instrumental in creating a stronger family unit which is able to plan for an uncertain future. The counselor's input may affect how the HIV-positive client shares the test results and communicates the need for further testing. The counselor needs to respect the client's perceptions about how the significant others will react while being clear that they have a right to know that they are at risk or may already have been infected.

An HIV-positive woman or man who has been infected by a sexual partner who was engaging in clandestine behaviors is often very upset. There may be a need to place blame and the counselor needs to assist the client in recognizing that this is a common initial reaction. It may help to role-play the first meeting with the significant other. If the relationship has been meeting each person's needs, then the counselor should support its continuance. The counselor needs to be aware of any personal values and beliefs which may be imposed on the client. For example, a female counselor may identify with a woman who contracted HIV infection from her husband of 5 years. In expressing feelings that the situation is "unfair," the counselor may agree and express angry sentiments towards the client's husband. This reaction, while honest, will not contribute to the therapeutic relationship.

It is very upsetting for a mother to think that she has transmitted HIV infection to her young child. If the female HIV-positive client has children under 6 years of age, they need to be tested for the virus. The initial response to this suggestion is often horror that the children, who look healthy, may actually be infected by HIV. It is probably helpful to schedule a separate appointment for the children so that the mother is not faced with learning her child's HIV status at the same time that she is processing information about her own health status. If a child older than 6 years of age has a positive HIV reaction, then perinatal transmission becomes less likely and child abuse should be thoroughly investigated. At this point, the counselor should consult with other providers, especially a social worker, who can assist with investigating possible sexual abuse.

Other topics also need to be discussed during the post-test session when the client is HIV positive. Helping a client to understand the difference between HIV infection and AIDS can be very challenging, but clients need to know where they are on the continuum. A diagnosis of AIDS, in contrast to one of HIV infection, has disability and other financial ramifications including possible eligibility for public assistance.

Self-help measures concerning nutrition, prevention of infection, overall health care, and the care of pets needs discussion. Ways to prevent transmission of the virus need to be strongly reinforced. Precautions to be taken with body fluids, especially blood, should be made clear to the client. Women need to know how to dispose of products used during menstruation. Referral to self-help groups such as Body Positive should be offered along with printed information. Clients should be counseled about alerting other health care providers to their HIV status. It should be pointed out that it is in the client's best interest to inform other health care providers so appropriate treatment interventions can be developed. The HIV-positive client must be referred to a primary care provider—physician or nurse—for treatment specific to HIV infection. The counselor should assist the client to identify the "next steps." These usually involve further blood testing and medications. Before the client leaves, a follow-up plan should be developed and appointments established.

SUMMARY

The skills of the health care provider engaged in HIV counseling will have an impact on the interaction with the client. As a nurse counselor, I have found that these clients draw on a myriad of professional and personal resources. Caring, respect, honesty, and the ability to recognize when to consult with other providers are essential characteristics of anyone doing HIV counseling. Client satisfaction and the incorporation of suggested behavior changes result from interaction with an interdisciplinary team whose members freely collaborate with one another and display these qualities.

REFERENCE

Burroughs Wellcome Co. 1988. *The Diagnosis and Management of HIV Disease: A Reference Manual.* New York: World Health Communications, Inc. (Obtainable from World Health Communications, Inc., 41 Madison Ave., New York, NY 10010.)

8

Organic Mental Syndromes Secondary to HIV Infection of the Central Nervous System

Ivan K. Goldberg, MD

In about 10% of AIDS patients the presenting complaint will be the symptoms of a HIV-induced organic mental disorder (Wortis 1986). The early symptoms of AIDS dementia are commonly attributed to reactive depression or misconstrued as concomitants of systemic illness (Navia and Price 1986). When there are questions about the presence of AIDS-related encephalopathy, the picture may be clarified by the use of magnetic resonance imaging (MRI), which may demonstrate extensive unequivocal diffuse white matter disease causing enlarged ventricles (Shabas, Gerard, Cunha et al. 1987). The organic mental disorders caused by AIDS include:

1. *Dementia.* Global cognitive impairment with undisturbed consciousness is found in patients with dementia. Early complaints by patients with AIDS dementia include:
   a. malaise, apathy and/or fatigue
   b. decreased memory and concentration
   c. psychomotor slowing
   d. heightened sensitivity to alcohol and other drugs
   e. weakness in the legs or problems with gait
   f. hypersomnia
   g. social withdrawal
2. *Amnesic syndromes.* In patients with HIV-induced amnesic syndrome there is impairment in short- and long-term memory which is *not* accompanied by reduced ability to maintain and shift attention (as in delirium) or impairment in abstract thinking, judgment, or other disturbances of higher cortical function as in dementia.

3. *Personality changes.* Patients with AIDS encephalopathy may show signs of an organic personality disorder. As pointed out in the DSM-IIIR, affective instability, recurrent outbursts of aggression or rage, markedly impaired social judgment, marked apathy and indifference, or suspiciousness or para- noid ideation are common symptoms of such a personality disorder.

4. *Anxiety and mood disorders.* Recurrent panic attacks or anxiety caused by HIV infection of the central nervous system (CNS) are found in patients with HIV-caused organic anxiety reac- tions. Patients with HIV-induced organic mood syndrome show a prominent and persistent depressed, elevated or expansive mood, resembling either a manic episode or a major depressive episode. Such organic mood syndromes may be the initial symptom caused by HIV infection (Kermani, Borod, Brown et al. 1985).

5. *Psychotic manifestations.* Prominent delusions, and prominent persistent or recurrent hallucinations caused by HIV infection of the CNS are the major symptoms of organic delusional syn- drome and organic hallucinosis, respectively.

6. *Mistakes in diagnosis.* It must be remembered that the cognitive, motor, and behavioral manifestations may be the initial symp- toms of AIDS and frequently appear at a time when the patient is medically well (Beckett et al. 1987). Such CNS symptoms may be the *only* evidence of HIV infection. The human immu- nodeficiency virus has its own intrinsic tropism for the ner- vous system, resulting sometimes in acute encephalopathic syndromes and often in a pattern of progressive dementia reminiscent of Alzheimer's disease (Osborn, 1986).

COURSE AND OUTCOME

The earliest symptoms of the AIDS dementia complex usually are im- paired memory and concentration with psychomotor slowing. Early motor deficits commonly seen included ataxia, leg weakness, tremor, and loss of fine motor coordination; while the behavioral disturbances most commonly seen were apathy and withdrawal, but occasionally a frank organic psychosis and/or an affective disorder were seen. Seizures may also be the earliest indicators of HIV infection of the CNS (Uldry, Steck, Regli et al. 1987). It is important to differentiate between the early signs of AIDS dementia, particularly, decreased acuity, slowed mentation, psychomotor retardation and the early signs of a depression. In the most advanced stages of the illness, patients exhibit a stereotyped picture of severe dementia, mutism, incontinence, paraplegia, and in some cases myoclonus.

Ayers, Abrams, and Newell (1987), using neuropsychological testing, demonstrated that neuropsychological deficits may be found in 27% of individuals with AIDS-related complex (ARC) compared to none in a normal control group. ARC also may present as a paranoid psychosis (Beckett, Summergrad, Manschreck et al. 1987; Halevie-Goldman, Potkin, and Poyourow 1987) and clinicians should be aware that dementia or psychosis may be the presenting symptoms of both ARC and AIDS (Navia and Price 1987; Bach and Boothby 1986). Since such individuals may be seronegative and since it may take much time before they develop more typical symptoms, it is important to look for evidence of HIV infection in the cerebral spinal fluid (CSF).

The magnitude of the AIDS dementia problem may be appreciated when it is remembered that approximately 60% of adult AIDS patients eventually develop dementia (Barnes 1986; Wortis 1986). In at least one series, 100% of children aged 10 months to 5 years with AIDS, involvement of the CNS was documented clinically, radiologically, and/or electro-physiologically in all patients (Ultmann et al. 1985).

Children with AIDS are not spared neuropsychiatric complications. As in adults, the CNS effects of AIDS may be the first manifestation of HIV infection. AIDS should be suspected or excluded in children at increased risk for AIDS presenting with either acquired atypical CNS infection or unexplained developmental regression, even in the absence of other clinical symptoms of pediatric AIDS (Biggemann, Voit, Neuen et al. 1987). As pediatric AIDS patients manifest variable neurodevelopmental courses, rehabilitative intervention services must be tailored to meet individual needs (Ultmann, Diamond, Ruff et al. 1987).

ETIOLOGY OF NEUROBEHAVIORAL MANIFESTATIONS

Infection of the Brain by HIV

Subacute encephalitis is the most common cause of altered behavior in patients with AIDS (Gabuzda and Hirsch 1987). Such subacute encephalitis causes progressive cognitive, motor, and behavioral abnormalities in about two-thirds of AIDS patients at some point in their illness. Demyelination, gliosis of the gray and white matter, focal necrosis, microglial nodules, atypical oligodendrocyte nuclei, and multinucleation of cells have been reported in up to 90% of autopsied patients with AIDS (de la Monte, Ho, Schooley et al. 1987). It has been demonstrated that HIV enters the brain during the earliest stages of infection. A degree of tropism for monocyte/macrophages and possibly for cells within the CNS seems certain (McArthur 1987). As it is unlikely that presently available treatments for AIDS will eliminate HIV from the central nervous system (CNS), there exists a possibility that over the next few years many of the 2 to 3 million individuals already infected with HIV will show dementia or other HIV-associated neuropsychiatric disorders. This poses severe psychological, social, and legal problems for individuals at risk to develop AIDS, their families and friends, and for society as a whole. The neuropsychiatric manifestations of AIDS can occur as sequelae of opportunistic infections, of AIDS-associated neoplastic processes (primary lymphomas of the brain, Kaposi's sarcoma), or of the retrovirus itself (Negele and Kaschka 1987). Aseptic meningitis may also be caused.

Opportunistic CNS Infection

Toxoplasmosis is the most commonly observed CNS infection in AIDS patients, other than CNS infection with HIV itself. The toxoplasmosis causes a diffuse encephalopathy or space-occupying and necrotic lesions. Fever, confusion, and focal neurological manifestations are the main clinical manifestations (Leport, Vilde, Katlama et al. 1987). As opposed to the more usual forms of toxoplasmosis, the serological diagnosis is unreliable and the therapeutic response in most cases is poor. Other sources of CNS infection include cytomegalovirus, cryptococcosis, herpes zoster encephalomyelitis, atypical mycobacteria, Candida, and progressive multifocal leukoencephalopathy.

PATHOLOGY

Less than 10% of the brains of individuals dying of AIDS are histologically normal. Abnormalities are found predominantly in the white matter and in the subcortical structure, with relative sparing of the cortex. In both adults and children with AIDS dementia who are seronegative, the HIV may be found in the CSF (Shaw et al. 1985). Using monoclonal antibodies, Pumarola, Navia, and Cordon (1987) detected infection in white matter and basal ganglia in a distribution paralleling that of the major neuropathological abnormalities. Viral antigen was identified principally in perivascular and parenchymal macrophages and in multinucleated cells of macrophage origin.

TREATMENT

AZT may be useful in reversing some of the symptoms of HIV-associated neurobehavioral abnormalities. Patients with HIV-related dementia may show improvement as assessed by clinical examination, psychometric tests, nerve conduction studies, and PET scans. Peptide T may prevent GP-120, a glycoprotein on the coat of the HIV, from damaging neurons.

REFERENCES

Ayers, M.R., D.I. Abrams, I.G. Newell et al. 1987. Performance of individuals with AIDS on the Luria-Nebraska neuropsychological battery. *Int. J. Clin. Neuropsychol.* 9:101–105.

Bach, M.C., and J.A. Boothby. 1986. Dementia associated with human immuno-deficiency virus with a negative ELISA. *N. Engl. J. Med.* 315: 891–892.

Barnes, D.M. 1986. AIDS-related brain damage unexplained. *Science* 232:1091–1093.

Beckett, A., P. Summergrad, T. Manschreck et al. 1987. Symptomatic HIV infection of the CNS in a patient without clinical evidence of immune deficiency. *Am. J. Psychiatry* 144:1342–1344.

Biggemann, B., T. Voit, E. Neuen et al. 1987. Neurological manifestations in three German children with AIDS. *Neuropediatrics* 18:99–106.

Halevie-Goldman, B.D., S.G. Potkin and P. Poyourow. 1987. AIDS-related complex presenting as psychosis. *Am. J. Psychiatry* 144:964.

Kermani, E.J., J.C. Borod, P.H. Brown et al. 1985. New psychopathologic findings in AIDS: case report. *J. Clin. Psychiatry* 46:240–241.

Leport, C., J.L. Vilde, C. Katlama et al. 1987. Toxoplasmose cerebrale de l'immunodeprime: diagnostic et traitement. *Ann. Med. Intern.* 138:30–33.

McArthus, J.C. 1987. Neurologic manifestations of AIDS. *Medicine* 66: 407–437.

Navia, B.A. and R.W. Price. 1986. Dementia complicating AIDS. *Psychiat. Ann.* 16:158–166.

Navia, B.A. and R.W. Price. 1987. The acquired immunodeficiency syndrome dementia complex as the presenting or sole manifestation of human immunodeficiency virus infection. *Arch. Neurol.* 44:65–69.

Negele, J. and W.P. Kaschka. 1987. Das erworbene Immundefektsyndrom (AIDS). *Fortschr. Neurol. Psychiatr.* 55:205–222.

Osborn, J.E. 1986. AIDS and the world of the 1990s: here to stay. *Aviat. Space Environ. Med.* 57:1208–1214.

Shabas, D., G. Gerard, R. Cunha et al. 1987. MRI appearance of AIDS subacute encephalopathy. *Comput. Radiol.* 11:69–73.

Shaw, G.M. et al. 1985. HTLV-III infection in brains of children and adults with AIDS encephalopathy. *Science* 227:177–182.

Uldry, P.A., A.J. Steck, F. Regli et al. 1987. Complications neurologiques accompagnant le syndrome d'immunodeficience acquise (SIDA): Etude d'un collectif de 8 cas. *Schweiz. Med. Wochenschr.* 117:560–569

Ultmann, M.H. et al. 1985. Developmental abnormalities in infants and children with acquired immune deficiency syndrome (AIDS) and AIDS-related complex. *Devlop. Med. Child. Neurol.* 27:563–571.

Wortis, J. 1986. Neuropsychiatry of acquired immune deficiency syndrome. *Biol. Psychiatry* 21:1357-1359.

9

Psychotherapeutic Management of an HIV-Positive Patient

Seymour E. Coopersmith, EdD

Mark, a 35-year-old divorced lawyer living in New York City, called for an appointment for therapy to treat his intense anxiety. He was referred by a colleague of mine who was treating a good friend of his and, consequently, would experience a conflict of interest treating both Mark and his friend. My colleague was also aware that I was interested in treating AIDS-related cases. When Mark called, he related that 2 days before he had tested positive for HIV and that he was extremely anxious. On the phone he related that the previous night he had had a dream in which he had lost both of his arms in an accident, and said, "I thought you might be interested in knowing about that." He wanted to know if I was familiar with AIDS-related problems, and whether I thought I could "handle" him and his problems. He said it was urgent that I see him as soon as possible, so I scheduled an appointment with him for the following day.

The next day when I came out to greet Mark in the waiting room of my office I could feel his anxiety. He was a tall, handsome, well-dressed man with wavy blond hair. He put down his briefcase, in a perfunctory, businesslike fashion, and proceeded to tap his foot anxiously as he told me his story:

Life had recently been going well for him, both personally and professionally. He was engaged to be married and was under consideration for a partnership in his law firm, where he specialized in corporate law. This was after a failed marriage and years of struggle in a prior law firm that did not, he felt, appreciate his efforts and ability. Though life had been a struggle, he had never been in therapy because he felt it could be a "crutch" and he wanted to be able to solve his problems on his own.

About a year prior to his first session with me, he had had an affair with a young paralegal, named Jill, who worked in his office. At first, they both resisted the idea of a relationship because they didn't want to "contaminate" their professional interaction. After a series of lunches and dinners, however, their contacts became more romantic. Jill was ambitious, hoping that she might one day go to law school herself. Her blue-collar background was in stark contrast with Mark's upper middle-class upbringing. Jill's two brothers and an uncle were New York City policemen, accustomed to wearing their revolvers around the house. Jill still lived at home with her parents and two brothers, and after several months of dating, invited Mark to her home in Brooklyn. Mark, who was Jewish, was accepted into Jill's Irish Catholic home, though with some reservation. One of Jill's brothers was antagonistic to Mark, and said to Jill, "Why do you want to date one of them? He's not like us." Mark himself was "put off by their blue-collar mentality." He was particularly annoyed by her brothers' sarcastic, homophobic sense of humor. Mark didn't tell his parents that he was dating someone "out of the faith" because he knew from past experience that they would be hostile to the idea.

Shortly after Mark and Jill began to date, they had a talk about sex, AIDS, and their experiences with other partners. Jill wanted to know if Mark had been tested for AIDS. He minimized her concern, telling her he had been very discreet and had only had a few sexual encounters since his divorce 4 years earlier. All of them, he assured her, were with "very nice girls." Jill told Mark that since her graduation from college she had only been with one man because, as she put it, she had little time for men. Since she had not been sexually "intimate" with a man for 3 years, she assumed that she was not at risk for AIDS. Neither of them were, in fact, particularly well informed about AIDS or the contagious potential of an AIDS-related viral infection. She was adamant, however, that he be tested prior to sexual intercourse because he had been with many more potential disease carriers. Human nature, however, was more powerful than her cautious resolve. Within a month after they began dating, they began having frequent "non-safe" sexual intercourse, as well as oral sex. A few months later she developed a vaginal infection and began questioning Mark about any prior sexual involvements which might have led to her being infected by Mark. She insisted that he have a blood test. He reluctantly agreed. Two weeks before he came to see me, he had gone for a blood test and, at the recommendation of the physician, agreed to be tested for AIDS at the same time.

The tests came back indicating that he was HIV positive. He was, initially, hysterical and distraught. He then went to a public health center where he was assured that the results would remain confidential. He was retested and again the results came back HIV positive.

Meanwhile, Jill's vaginal infection had cleared up and Mark had told her that he had tested negative for her infection. He did not tell her, however, that he was HIV positive.

Mark felt anxious and guilty. He was afraid he might have infected Jill with the virus and would be responsible for her death. But he was even more afraid that her brothers would kill him if they found out that he had infected her with the AIDS virus. These anxieties compounded his sense of misery about his own condition and his sense of foreboding about his foreshortened future.

When I asked Mark how he thought he might have gotten the virus, he at first suggested it might have come from a prostitute with whom he had spent an evening. At the same time, he protested that he was not homosexual, even though I hadn't raised the issue with him. When I mentioned this fact, he got defensive and suggested that he just wanted to clear the air about any ideas I might have about his being homosexual. In light of this discussion, I asked him if he had ever been an intravenous (IV) drug user. He became irate and said that maybe this wasn't the right kind of therapy for him—that he might be better off with a psychiatrist who at least had a medical background and could better advise him about his condition. I told him that I was interested in knowing more about how he might have gotten infected to better understand him and his lifestyle. This made him even more defensive, but after several more sessions he confessed to having had some homosexual activity. He claimed it was over 15 years ago, so "it couldn't possibly have had anything to do with my HIV infection." He explained that at that time he subscribed to bisexuality as a political statement, but that he considered himself heterosexual. He said he had been "curious" about homosexuality, but assured me that he was then and always would be heterosexual.

During our twice-weekly sessions Mark was anxious and distrustful of me. He did not want anyone to know that he was HIV positive. I suggested to him that he was afraid that I might reveal that he was infected. He agreed that it wasn't logical, but he just didn't want anyone to know that he was seeing me. He was also afraid of making me angry for fear that I would take revenge on him in some way. I pointed out to him that his fear that people would take revenge on him might be part of a more pervasive anxiety he had about making people angry. After some discussion, he felt more relaxed with me, and less anxious about Jill's brothers attacking and killing him.

He continued to read voraciously about AIDS, and spent a good deal of time during his sessions talking about AIDS and the articles he had been reading. He alternated between the idea that heterosexual transmission was not a proven factor and his dread that Jill was already infected. He also alternated between guilt and fear. At times he would take full responsibility for his dilemma; at other times, he would blame everyone but himself. My objective was to help him to understand the difference between blame and responsibility—and if he couldn't help feeling guilty, to determine if there was anything that he could do to alleviate his guilt. I also wanted to help him to understand the conflict between his conscience and his fear, and to consider the reality of this conflict, as well as any unconscious ramifications. In addition I wanted to help him with the reality of his life, supportively, and cognitively. To the extent possible, I tried to help him deal with what might be inevitable, his death within several years, taking into consideration the possibility that medical advances would intervene such that HIV-positive infection did not have to translate into AIDS.

Mark's fear of death, and his helplessness to do anything about the idea, if not the reality, that he would eventually get AIDS and die, were pervasive in the early months of treatment. At times, he would pleadingly extend his arms, palms upward, with tears in his eyes, and ask, "Why me?" He wanted me to save him, somehow.

Initially, I was caught up in his wish to be saved. My sense that it was my job to do just that caused me a great deal of anxiety. When I became aware of the reason for my intense reactions to his quandary, how his needs coalesced with my own inner wishes to save him, I could then tell him that, realistically, I couldn't save him, but I could help him. He questioned the value of any help other than changing his morbid situation and giving him "another chance." Rationally he understood what I was saying, but emotionally he felt it was intolerable. After several months of supportive psychotherapy, we established an alliance and he developed a more trusting attitude. He began to accept the idea that he needed to learn more about himself so that he could decide how to live his life. Then more of the truth came out.

About 3 years before he came into treatment, he was having an affair with a woman whom he was considering marrying. He was, however, relatively unexcited by the sex life he was having with this woman, but felt it was unethical to have sex with any other women while he was seeing her. One day, he wandered into a gay bar in lower Manhattan, "out of curiosity." He was standing at the bar, having a drink, when a man came over and started talking to him. Mark told him that he was "straight," but that he was curious about gay life. The man asked Mark if he had ever had a homosexual experience. When Mark mentioned his homosexual college experience, the other man said that he too had had some homosexual experiences earlier in life. Mark felt a kinship with the man and accepted an invitation to go back to his apartment for a drink. They had drinks there, and laughingly began to exchange fantasies of what they would do or want done if they were to have a homosexual experience. They ended up having anal intercourse, without protection, with Mark as the recipient. Mark felt at the time that as long as he didn't put his penis into the other man that he was safe from infection and "not really homosexual." This was just the first of many such episodes, with this man and many others. He found these experiences, and wandering into Manhattan bars to seek out just the right man, far more stimulating and exciting than sex with women. Yet, during this entire period he maintained that he was "just fooling around," and that he was clearly heterosexual. As the anal recipient, he felt he was experiencing a "fullness" that he didn't experience with women. It was, in his mind, a more liberated sense of sexuality. This was the first time he revealed this secret aspect of his life to someone other than a sexual partner. Mark felt quite relieved that he could be more open, but he didn't feel relieved about his dilemma. He insisted that he was heterosexual, continued to struggle with the conflict between his conscience and his fear, and was intensely anxious that he would develop symptoms of ARC or AIDS (i.e., he was constantly taking his temperature, both literally and figuratively).

Because he was "split" in his choice of sexual interest, he had maintained a duality of homosexual trysts and heterosexual dating. He was exited about the idea of being with men and identified with the idea of being with women. The latter interest was so great that it belied the idea that his heterosexual interests were a defense against his homosexual wishes. When he started to become involved with Jill, he stopped visiting the gay pick-up spots.

Mark was blind to the pathological or unconscious implications of his behavior. He rationalized extensively, suggesting that behavior doesn't need to reflect one's true self. The treatment, at this early time, was geared to providing the support he needed to deal with his overwhelming anxiety. The treatment was also an attempt to forge a therapeutic alliance which would allow for the development of an increasingly trusting treatment relationship, and the transformation of the treatment process into a developmental, insight-oriented process which would help him to understand the nature of his conflicts.

Mark's reaction to his anxiety about AIDS and ultimately death was a function of reality perception and unconscious anxieties. When he talked about dying, he wanted me not to confirm his certitude that AIDS was inevitable. We discussed the literature each of us had read, particularly regarding the latest statistics of the probability of an HIV-positive person evolving to the ARC or AIDS stages. We also spent considerable time considering his becoming involved in experimental drug treatment programs, as well as discussing the importance of good diet and good physical conditioning. Though the latter may seem superficial to some, this kind of communication provided him with a supportive base which counteracted his pervasive sense of helplessness and hopelessness. It gave him the feeling that he could be active in the quest for survival. At times, however, he was over-whelmed with the conviction that he was going to die. I usually responded to this reaction with the suggestion that it was much too soon for him to take such a position; that research and development were moving rapidly in the direction of drugs that might inhibit or prevent an HIV-positive condition from developing into AIDS.

If Mark had AIDS, I might then be confronted with the conflict of whether to confirm that it was likely that he would die soon or, as the case may be, to support his denial and struggle for survival against the overwhelming probability that it would be to no avail. Kübler-Ross (1987), for example, advocates the confrontational approach and a hospice attitude towards death and dying. She suggests that AIDS patients should accept the inevitable so that they can die with dignity and a sense of communal value. Matt, Sementilli, and Burish (1988) suggest that denial (of death) can be valuable as a coping mechanism. This suggests the support of denial as a defense, rather than its anal-ysis. But with Mark, this consideration was, I believe, premature. When someone is actually dying of AIDS, the goals of treatment are radically at variance with the goals of treatment of someone who may die of AIDS. Intrinsically, my interventions with Mark were geared to help him understand that his anxiety was not only reality-based, but that there was also a value in coming to terms with the fear of death, and that he, like anyone else who comes into treatment, has to learn to accept the reality of death to be able to face life. Finally, regarding his death anxiety, I pointed out that we needed to differentiate between anxiety that is reality-based and death-anxiety which may be part of his overall anxiety (i.e., childhood fears arising from develop-mental problems).

My difficulty in establishing a therapeutic alliance was traceable to his intense anxiety, and his insistence that nothing was more important than the anxiety about whether he would live or die. Consequently, he was consistently trying to enlist me either as an information-provider or a savior. He resisted the idea that we might work together to help him understand himself and make changes conducive to conflict-resolution. To some extent, in order to give him what I thought was necessary support, I did not oppose his resistance.

However, when his paranoid anxiety level was reduced, I would interpret his resistance as transference anxiety. I pointed out to him that we were doing as much as we could about the reality of his viral infection, but that we also needed to attend to his life. For this reason, although I was only seeing him (sitting up) twice a week, I encouraged him to remember his dreams and fantasies. Interestingly, his dreams were not involved with AIDS or death anxiety; they were involved with sexual issues and unresolved preoedipal conflicts. His fear of trusting me, or anyone, for that matter, made the development of a therapeutic alliance difficult.

The movement toward a more insight-oriented therapy, which was directed to unconscious, as well as conscious, processes, was aided considerably by my discussions with Joyce McDougall, who stressed the need to understand and analyze the resistive patterns. This case was discussed, during its early stages, in a group setting, with McDougall as a consultant. We worked toward the goal of understanding specific treatment problems, as well as countertransferential factors that are sometimes more discernible in a professional communication. McDougall stressed the importance of orienting the treatment toward a therapeutic structure which would help the patient understand the need to focus on his life, not his death. The coalescence of his anxiety and his resistance had been making this difficult.

The transference anxieties that manifested themselves in this early phase of treatment seemed to be oriented around the wish for a strong father figure, as well as anxiety about the development of a homosexual transference. Mark had a tendency to withold the therapy payment we had agreed on in the contract we'd established, because he said he needed the money for a new sports car. When he was confronted with the superficiality of this expressed wish in comparison with the importance of therapy, he would pay his bill. At other times he sought to test me for corruptibility by suggesting that it might be better for me if he paid me in cash, and that he wanted to know my preference.

He was also anxious about what he might learn about his relationship with his mother and with women in general and how this might impact on his relationship with Jill. The details of his early life that he shared with me were sketchy because he insisted on focusing on his condition. He described an intense love-hate relationship with his mother. He was vague about his father and described him as being "a nice guy." But it soon became clear that he had been seeking out a father figure in his homosexual activity so that he might get from others what he didn't get from his father. When he talked about women in general, he revealed an underlying hostility. We considered whether his anxiety that he might have infected Jill might not in some way be related to a need to protect her against his aggressive impulses toward her as well as toward other women. This was brought out not as an alternative to the reality-oriented anxiety that he might have infected her, but as an adjunctive motive which might help him understand the depth and intensity of his fears. In the discussion about his aggression, he remembered the dream that he had had the night before he first came to see me. In this dream, he said, "someone came up behind me and cut off both my arms." Perhaps, we considered, he felt he would be better off with his hands cut off—then he would not be able to hurt anyone. The implications for self-castration seemed obvious, but were left for a future interpretation when his characterological style could be considered. At these times, he was more anxious about what he might have done to Jill than he was about his own death. He would ask with despair, "What have I done?" I tried to help him understand that his anxiety about hurting women existed before the viral infection anxiety.

He struggled against the idea of treatment whenever we touched on anything related to hostility towards women or to homosexuality, asking "Where is this going to get us?" Since, however, this is a treatment case-in-progress, which is substantially disguised in order to protect the privacy and anonymity of the patient, I cannot be more specific about some of the details of his life. Nor can I reveal the current status of the case to any greater degree than has already been presented.

The countertransference factors that have influenced my work with Mark were substantial during the first few months. There were times when I felt quite anxious and other times when I was either depressed or angry at him. My early anxiety was related to a conflict between my wish to save him (a personal countertransference issue), and the realization that I was, in fact, quite helpless. When I became aware of this anxiety, I was able to direct him to the reality that I could not save him, but I might be able to help him. Early on, I found myself washing my hands after a session with Mark, particularly after the first session when he shook hands with me at the end of the session. When I became aware of this compulsive act and considered my anxiety about transmission, particularly in relation to his homosexual transference, the behavior stopped. I have since learned that this is not an uncommon reaction for therapists who are treating HIV-positive or AIDS patients.

There were times when Mark induced depression or guilt feelings in me. This happened at times when he was most anxious and accusatory about my not helping, that is, saving him from death or being murdered by Jill's family. Once I was aware that this was a product of his anxiety, I was able to point out to him that his anxiety about his feelings of helplessness made him insist that I (a much stronger man) should do for him what he couldn't do for himself. When treatment moved in the direction of insight-oriented discovery of his unconscious motives, his transference anxiety and my countertransferential anxieties were substantially diminished. For example, when he was able to understand that he was viewing his viral infection as a payback for forbidden sexual desires and activities, he became less anxious and less accusatory. Likewise, homophobic anxieties were viewed as countertransferentially induced homosexual transference manifestations. He gradually eased up on his insistence that our relationship was strictly professional, and he accepted the idea that personal feelings might enter into our work together. He reached the point where he could verbalize positive, though not erotic, feelings toward me, as well as feelings of gratitude.

One final issue of countertransference that emerged involved my anxiety about Jill as it related to my legal and moral obligations. I felt she needed to know that she might be infected with HIV, for herself as well as for others. There were several issues that I looked at that were germane to this conflict. First, I felt I should consider whether Jill was, in fact, in any danger. The evidence was inconclusive, but the data about heterosexual infection indicate a strong likelihood of infection when intercourse takes place between a woman and a bisexual man. This potential is enhanced with repeated exposure. The logistics of informing Jill were quite difficult, if not impossible, because I did not know Jill's name or the name of Mark's firm, and I felt it would be devious to try to get this information from Mark, but I did not have any other resource for this information. Still, all of this was overshadowed by the question of whether any efforts should be made in this direction, regardless of whether it was logistically possible.

Second, as a psychoanalyst, I come from a tradition where the privacy and anonymity of a patient's communications are considered sacred even though they may conflict with the rights and needs of society. Third, I felt there was a distinction that needed to be made between the duty to protect Mark and the duty to inform Jill. Was Jill currently in danger, or not? Since Mark had acted in good conscience, immediately, upon learning of his diagnosis, and engaged only in safe sex with Jill, she was apparently no longer in any new danger of infection. In other words, if she was by this time HIV positive, then it was after the fact. Since she was not having sex with anyone else, the risk of further spread of the contagion was not a problem. Consequently, it was my belief that she was protected, but not informed.

Finally, I considered the legal and moral implications of this dilemma in light of *Tarasoff* v. *Regents of the University of California* (1976). At the time of the writing of this case study, the application of Tarasoff to the threat of HIV infection has not yet been litigated in the appellate courts, according to Gary B. Melton, who evaluated "Ethical and Legal Issues in AIDS-Related Practice" in an article in the November, 1988 issue of the *American Psychologist*. According to Melton, firm conclusions have not yet been drawn. The Tarasoff ruling indicates that the therapist "incurs an obligation to use reasonable care to protect the intended victim against (such) danger." If, however, a seropositive patient has already had infection-potential sex with someone, the danger has already taken place. It is, therefore, after the fact, although we might agree that it is not a risk that should be indemnified by continued sexual risk-taking. As indicated previously, the psychoanalytic model of patient-therapist interaction is committed to the confidentiality of patient communications. Consequently, any betrayal of this commitment runs the risk of a breakdown of trust in the treatment matrix. An alternative, however, raises the question of whether the therapist can accomplish the same goal by making interventions that would help the patient to understand his dilemma, and to decide what alternatives might be satisfactory to his reasonable conscience. A more psychopathic or sociopathic personality would be less likely to be in treatment in the first place (Coopersmith 1981) and, therefore, outside of the realm of a treatment problem.

Along the same lines, Melton points out that "even if Tarasoff extends to risk of HIV infection, it does not necessarily require warning the potential 'victims' (e.g., sexual partners) of infected clients. Other action may suffice if a therapist reasonably believes that an HIV-infected client is not following authoritative risk reduction practices and is engaging in sexual intercourse without use of condoms or is sharing unsterilized needles with unsuspecting partners" (Melton 1988).

Following his diagnosis, Mark had quickly determined to take all precautions not to infect anyone else. In this case, the cost to society of breach of confidentiality, might far exceed the benefits because it might polarize the patient away from the limited trust he developed and perhaps lead him into violations of self and others, in a world he perceives as uncaring and untrustworthy. In this regard, "Undeniably, there is special sensitivity in discussion of an individual's sexual practices and drug-taking history. Public knowledge about either can subject the client to embarrassment, social stigma, and criminal penalties. Relationships between health professionals and the groups most directly affected by AIDS often have been tenuous and breaches of confidentiality would be likely to intensify such mistrust and to deter individuals from seeking treatment or counseling" (Melton 1988). In a world which is moving in the direction of an AIDS epidemic, the mental health profession needs to be an important resource for therapy based on confidentiality and trust.

Although there have not been any decisions about the application of Tarasoff to HIV infection, this does not mean that individual states may not take action to require clinicians to breach confidentiality under local public health authority. In this case, though, any attempts to notify Jill by anyone other than Mark would assume that she has been infected, although it has not been established, would certainly destroy Mark's therapy, and possibly put Mark in grave jeopardy. Summarily, then, we are dealing, on this issue, with complex clinical, social, and moral issues which may best be decided, at this time, on an individual, case-by-case basis.

SUMMARY AND CONCLUSIONS

The treatment of an HIV-positive patient invokes the need to employ unique parameters in psychoanalytically oriented psychotherapy. The need to be supportive and help the patient face the dilemma of possibly getting AIDS and dying is the first objective of treatment. It is essential, however, to help the patient move in the direction of living and away from the preoccupation with death. The orientation of treatment then depends on the pathological structures of the patient and the way in which the therapist would ordinarily treat such a patient.

The problem of dealing with social issues is one that remains unresolved. It appears, at this time, that it is more important to protect the confidentiality and anonymity of the patient than to expose the patient and create a circumstance in which he would lose all trust for the mental health profession. The future of this problem depends, to some degree, on the influence the mental health profession can have on social, ethical, and legal forces.

REFERENCES

Coopersmith, S.E. 1981. Object-instinctual and developmental aspects of perversion. *Psychiatry Rev.* 68:3, 371–383.

Gang, V. and N. Rudnick, eds. 1981. *AIDS: Facts and Issues.* New Brunswick, NJ: Rutgers University Press.

Kübler-Ross, E. 1987. *AIDS: The Ultimate Challenge.* New York: Macmillan.

Matt, D., M. Sementilli, and T. Burish. 1988. Denial as a strategy for coping with cancer. *J. Mental Health Counseling* 10:2.

McDougall, J. Personal communication.

Melton, G.B. 1988. Ethical and legal issues in AIDS-related practice. *Am. Psychologist* (November).

10

Going Public: An Interview

Karyn Teufel and Florence E. Selder, RN, PhD

Florence: What was it like for you to find out that you tested positive for HIV?

    Karyn: It was early May and I was ready to go to work and the phone rang. It was someone from the state health department telling me that one of my former lovers recommended me for testing. The woman couldn't tell me who it was. She just told me that a former lover had AIDS and recommended me for testing. My response was disbelief. It was like I was in a fog and I was just going through the motions and that as soon as I got tested I would find out that I'm negative and everything would go back to normal. There was no panic or anything. I really felt confident that I wasn't infected. Two weeks later I went back for the test results and Brenda, the nurse, came into the room with me. I knew from the look on her face that it was not going to be good news. And it wasn't. The three things I remembered from that meeting were: you tested positive; there is a confidentiality issue that you have to deal with, so don't go running out telling everybody because people have bizarre reactions to this; and, people do best if they reduce their stress. That last comment was almost comical because it created so much more stress. I left in a daze. I kept thinking, something has got to be wrong, this can't be right, this can't be real, I must have misunderstood, they're going to find out that the test was wrong, that it was a test error. The interesting thing about my keeping it confidential is that it was impossible. I ran into a friend of mine on my way out of the hospital, and when he kidded about having tested there and turned out negative, I just burst out crying and said I didn't. So I wasn't even out of the hospital when the pledge of confidentiality was already broken. I never could keep a secret. But to try and keep something like this confidential is ridiculous. The burden is too great. Nothing made sense to me for a long time. Even now, when I look at the statistics, only 4% of the people in our state with AIDS are women. Statistics take on a different meaning now. Here I am in that small 4%. At first, I didn't recognize the anger that I was feeling. I didn't know who to be mad at. I wasn't mad at the person who called the state. Because that relationship had been so long ago that neither of us knew what AIDS was. I don't believe I'd even heard the word back then. He was a real early contact after my marriage broke up. I never considered myself promiscuous, although I certainly wasn't virginal. He was, I believe, the second person I'd ever slept with after I separated from my husband.

Florence: How has AIDS changed you?

Karyn: I think it's like a new life. I'm having a hard time relating to anything non-AIDS. Nothing will ever be the same again. If they cured this disease tomorrow, and it all went away, I think that finding out that you're HIV positive is still a pivotal experience. Even if my condition cleared up and went away, I'm forever changed by that day. I got the news when I was 38. I'd been through a lot of other things in my life, and I had somehow managed to come through it all and to cope. I had plans for school and other things. Then, when I tested positive, I just couldn't seem to find the notion of a future. People dealing with terminal illnesses are told (and expected) to take it day to day. I had this future that might be. I didn't think I could cope, and I was very angry that I couldn't cope. All the guys in my support group seemed to be coping. After awhile, I started missing the old Karyn, the Karyn before the positive test. I was worried that she was gone forever, and there would never be that old Karyn again. It's only recently, within the past 6 months or so, that I've kind of taken the best from the old Karyn and put it with the new Karyn. How did my life change? I can't think, so many ways, and so many ways that I don't even realize yet. Somebody told me just the other day that HIV positive was giving me a gift, and that I am much wiser now. It occurred to me, what in the world am I going to do with all this wisdom? What's the point of being wise about things like this? The truth is, testing positive made me petty about a lot of things. I'd see a couple walking hand-in-hand in the park in the springtime, and I'd be angry at them. Why do they get to have that and I have to deal with this? Why is my love life over forever? I'm angry. Not having a love life is something that really bothers me. There are loneliness issues. It's like I've lost the ability to have sex, but I still have my sexuality. Everytime I have a sexual stirring, right away the old AIDS notion kicks in. I can't, and probably won't, ever have sex again, and it makes the fantasies harder to take. A lot of the guys in the support groups I go to are much younger than me. At least I've had my children. I've had 41 years, and some of these guys are 20 or 26 and they are dying already. That is tragic. If any one of them needed something from me, whether I liked them or not, I would do the best I could for him. In the beginning, I think one of the things I was afraid of was dying alone. If I'm not supposed to be telling anybody, and if none of my friends want to hear it, then it seemed as if I would be very lonely at the end. It was a neat thing to realize that we would all take care of each other.

Florence: How did your kids deal with it?

Karyn: It's hard to say. Dan was at a juvenile detention center when I told him, and I made sure that when I told him a counselor was there at the same time. I wanted Dan to know he'd have someone to go to and talk to about it. The counselor was very nice. We sat down and talked for quite a long time. She had as many questions as the kids did, because the available information is so bizarre. Some of it is inaccurate, some of it gives false hope, and some of it is true. The counselor took it very calmly and we talked to Dan about it for awhile. I really felt awful having to drop that on him, but I had to tell him. One of the reasons I had to tell him is that I decided I wasn't going to keep it a secret from anyone. I was going to do whatever I could do, public speaking, panel discussions, anything to help get the information out.

Florence: What made you decide to go public?

Karyn: Keeping it inside just didn't work for me. First of all, I think that it's nothing anyone should have to deal with—such an illness under all those circumstances.

Florence: What is it like when you're down?

Karyn: Helpless and hopeless. I think, why bother? When I was sick a couple of months ago, there were a lot of times I thought, why bother? So what. Just be sick and die and get it over with. Why prolong this? I don't see a future for myself other than just day to day, I don't want to say it's boring, but it doesn't seem very exciting. If you can't plan anything for the

future, it takes some of the spark out of things. There's
nothing to look forward to, except getting sicker and sicker.
There's nothing to look forward to, except all my terrific new
friends getting sicker and dying. How many deaths was I
going to have to see? Some of these guys have seen 10 to 12
funerals in the last 2 or 3 years. In some places in the bigger
cities it's even worse. You're going to funerals weekly. Sometimes more than once a week. With that as my future—just
watching my friends die around me and watching society
condemn us and shove us aside, I decided to do something.
The confidentiality issue was no longer an issue for me. I
thought, if I'm going to die, I'm not going to die nameless or
faceless. None of us deserves this. I didn't deserve this.
There are guys who have already died who refused to have
their last names used. It seems to me that we're all easy
enough to forget. When you know a person's full name and
address and you know something about that person, it's
harder to forget. All these people are dying and nobody
even knows it. I think that what is really sad is that even
after they're gone they don't want their last names used.
They don't want people to know that they had AIDS. I'm
angry at society for setting up conditions so it's this way.
People are so scared—to come out of the AIDS closet and the
gay closet, and of whatever else they're dealing with, that
they are dying without anybody knowing. There was a time
when I was almost suicidal, when I thought of just taking my
car up to the high-rise bridge, punching the gas, and going
over the edge—at least then I would go out somewhat spec-
tacularly. People would know my name and address, and
people who knew me would know what happened. The
notion of just quietly pulling into myself more and more,
and then dying without anybody knowing, bothers me a lot.
I've never been particularly afraid of dying and I don't think
I am now. But living with it is scary, and I worry about how
I'm going to finance this, and I wonder how am I or am I
going to be alone? It impacts every aspect of my life. I
couldn't prioritize. Everything seemed important, then
some counselors helped me to start pulling out what was
most important, what my major issues were, and what could
wait until a later time. That was a real breakthrough for me.
I was ready to lose my job because I'd gotten way behind on
my cab rent, and after I talked to the counselor for an hour,
she asked, "what do you need the most?" I said all I needed

was time. "How can you get more time?" she asked. I said I couldn't, but I could get my cab rent paid up so that I could continue to work. As long as I'm working at least I know I'm dealing with one of my control issues. I'm certainly not sick enough to quit working. I don't want to quit working. I need to work for a lot of different reasons and there I was on the brink of losing my job. I was afraid to look for a new job. I was having trouble with my memory. How could I learn a new job when I'm having trouble remembering some of the stuff I'm supposed to be doing on a job that I've had for 6 years? So I was afraid of losing my job, and then what I would do if I did. Since I've been able to prioritize again, my thinking is clearer. I've been feeling good since my thinking is clearer, and I'm able to plan things in advance.

Florence: What about the future?

Karyn: I have a more positive attitude now than I did before. There are a lot of good things coming out about the future. Dr. Salk has been doing some interesting research. They're not thinking of AIDS entirely as a fatal disease right now. They're thinking of it as more of a long-term illness, similar to diabetes or heart disease. With the proper monitoring and medication, we may have a longer lifespan than they originally thought. So that's encouraging. I don't feel quite as much doom and gloom. The only problem with it now is that people not in the AIDS community are sloughing it off. They tell me, "they're going to have a cure for that in no time, Karyn. You don't have anything to worry about anymore." The fact is, I don't have a lot of worries yet. A lot of my friends who are much sicker than I am are worried. Even if the predictions all come true, some of my friends are too sick, the disease is too far advanced, and even a cure won't help them. More populations of people will be coming down with it. More people are being infected and the numbers are rising. Even though some people are talking about cures and treatments, there are the IV drug users and teenagers starting to show up in these statistics. Kids! I know from my own experience that kids don't listen to this stuff. By nature, they don't pay a whole lot of attention to warnings. Life goes on forever and it's not going to happen to them. I couldn't convince them to have safe sex to avoid pregnancy, and now there's a much more serious reason for having safe sex and they're still just brushing it off. About the future, anytime somebody said, "Well, look on the bright side," I'd think, there is no bright side here. Don't be silly. I hear people say that good things have happened to them since this experience, but I haven't had many good things happen yet, other than the fact that the people I'm meeting are neat. I mean the guys that I was meeting with, and the people that were helping us. The people down at the AIDS project, the caliber of people that I started being with, really went way up. So that's kind of neat, and from that I sort of build on the good stuff. I really do think that I've got a decent future—whether or not I get it.

11

Facing the Diagnosis

Todd Butler and "Michael"

It is a special gift when a client is willing to share his thoughts and feelings so we may learn and improve our care.

Extrapolated from Todd's writings, this chapter provides an intimate glimpse into the days surrounding his being diagnosed HIV positive and his thoughts 2 years later. According to Todd's best friend, Michael, whose experience of Todd's life and death follows Todd's words, Todd wanted others to know what it was like to live with AIDS, to touch people's lives, and to change ignorance and fear into understanding.

TODD'S STORY

Finally, the 2-week waiting period is over. One o'clock this afternoon, mere hours before I get my results back from my antibody test and everyone will be able to relax. I don't know why everyone has been so shaken up. Sure, I was very ill for the entire month of October, but for me this is nothing out of the ordinary. I never have gotten a lot of colds and flu, but instead I usually get two long-term infections a year. They're usually seasonal, cold to warm weather. Besides, I've been living out in the country for over one year now, and before that in Milwaukee. This last year I've had a monogamous relationship, and let's face it, Wisconsin just isn't San Francisco or New York! I'd never even heard of AIDS until the television movie that was aired a couple of weeks ago.

Jesus Christ, they air a show on television about AIDS and my mother is right there thinking the worst. I'd swear martyrdom is a motherly instinct; always thinking the worst and always getting so excited. Oh well, 4 more hours and all this fuss will be finished.

Let me see now—vegetables, potatoes, turkey, sauces, pies, wine, and oh yes, can't forget champagne because tomorrow is Thanksgiving and reason to celebrate. Most of the family will be together, which is a miracle in itself. We can all celebrate my health!

Living out in the country has advantages as well as disadvantages. Getting to the hospital would take close to an hour, but with this weather and having to pick up Mom (she insisted on going with me) I decided to allot an extra half hour. The ride in was normal, with a lot of small talk about Thanksgiving, traffic, weather, and a new building going up. Mom seemed slightly tense and uneasy. I told her that even if the result was positive that it didn't mean I had AIDS, but just that I was exposed to the virus. This seemed to do the trick for her that moment, but it switched all the tension over to me. Now she is making small talk and I answer her, but without really listening. Now I'm wondering what if . . . I don't want to die . . . my God, what about all the people I could have given a death warrant to! I got a lump in my throat that actually burned going down. Then I thought—wait a minute! This can't be happening to me. . . .

While sitting in the waiting area, a million things started running through my mind. What a drab office. Do I have it? Finally, why am I waiting? Are they trying to find a way to tell me something I don't want to hear, and if they are, what am I going to tell Mom? Why did she wait in the car—was it "a mother's intuition"? All these confusing thoughts and all in a matter of seconds. My head felt like it was spinning. Then suddenly, as if applying an emergency brake, it stopped. The woman who took my blood greeted me and asked me to step into her office.

I entered her office and sat on a small sofa while she sat at her desk looking for my file—my results—my future! She looked over the file, which seemed to take minutes but I'm sure was just seconds. Here's that burning lump in my throat again. Then she got up from her desk and came over to sit beside me on the couch. This told me the results immediately. I knew I was dead.

Then she looked up at me with an expression like she was about to tell her best friend, "Your test came back positive." That sentence felt as if she were pointing a gun at me and had just pulled the trigger; that sentence was the bullet. No one has ever said anything to me that hurt so much. I remember she moved closer to me to explain that a positive result did not mean that I had AIDS. I had heard that before. Then we moved on to talking about precautions.

I listened. I didn't hear anything, but I listened. I had my own conversation going on in my mind. I don't want to die. Who else did I kill? Who am I killing? Why me, why am I being punished? How I wish I could just jump out of this filthy, lethal, infected body that used to be so slender and, as I'd been told, "cute"—now I hate it!

I did catch a few lines that held my attention for a moment. AIDS was not spread by casual contact. Casual contact? What's that? By this time, I was trembling on the inside, but not on the outside. The past 20 minutes seemed like seconds. By now my arms are full of "safe sex" information, doctor listings, phone numbers, and statistics. Statistics that would increase by at least one more at the next printing, I thought.

The nurse asked me if I had any questions, to which I replied, "No," still together on the outside. Then she asked if I wanted a hug. My answer was "no" for a number of reasons. I felt dirty, infected, and deadly, and I was afraid I would start to cry. She asked me if I would give her a hug, realizing, I'm sure, how I probably felt. So we hugged, she wished me luck, and I walked out.

Just outside the door, being alone for a mere instant started the tears, as though closing the door was the cue to begin. Just as fast as I began crying, I realized how long I had been in that room, and just how long I had left Mom sitting in the car, probably sweating bullets. What am I going to say to her? She has six kids and out of all of them, she and I have been the closest. I'd always tried to be there for her, all through my childhood. Always trying to fill in the gap left by my alcoholic stepfather who was never around. And she had been there for me. I think my being gay made our relationship special. Special in that she really had to learn to love the real me, not what most kids allow their parents to see. So now, how do I tell her that at the young age of 28, I'm going to die? Funny, she had always told me that she worried about how hard it would be on me when she died, and now I have to tell her that I'm going to die first.

I paused for a few moments to dry my eyes and get myself together, as well as to figure out what to say. I figured that there wasn't any easy way. But—if I told her the test came back positive but that it didn't mean I had, or ever would develop AIDS, and if I looked and sounded convincing—then she would be convinced. After that, I'd change the subject and everything would be okay.

Funny how things never work out as planned. I got into the car, said that everything was okay and just started driving off, trying to make it appear as though everything was alright. It just didn't work— or at least it didn't work well. As we were driving, I told her the test result and that I may never get sick. She seemed to buy it at the moment, but the next 35 minutes would seem never to pass. Not one word was spoken. I think we were both afraid to say a word for fear of falling apart. We were both too busy being strong for each other, not to mention being scared, and each of us was probably going through denial. After about 15 minutes of dealing with my emotions and all that was going through my mind, I felt like I was going to explode. I swallowed a lump in my throat that felt like it was the size of a grapefruit and as hot as lava. I needed to be alone in the worst way. However, to try to keep things going smoothly, I got off the freeway to finish my grocery shopping. I don't really believe it, but I think maybe she'll think that things aren't so bad—I mean, who goes shopping minutes after you've been told your life is over?

I was hoping that once we got inside the store things would go back to normal, but they didn't. I found myself trying to go down the different aisles, trying to find some space to be alone, even if just for a second. When I felt alone, I could hardly hold back the tears—kind of like having to go to the bathroom when you're just a mile or two away from home—but I also did not want to break down in the grocery store. Thank God I had a shopping list.

Back in the car, nothing changed. Still a total, dead silence, but at least there were only about 20 miles left to go. Once we got to Mom's house, I came in and helped her unpack her groceries. After unpacking, we turned and looked at each other, embraced, and started crying. All that we did was cry until there were no more tears left to cry. We spoke of how stupid we were being and how nothing could possibly happen to me. I gave her a hug and headed for home.

When I got into the car, I thought about driving down to the lake. I knew my sister would be at our home, and I really needed some time to myself. However, I knew the moment I walked out the door of Mom's house she would be on the phone calling Tammy. Her children had grown to be her only support system; she really doesn't have many friends, so we try to be there for her, just as she has always been there for us. So if I didn't go right home, she would just become upset. Normally, I would expect her to understand, but during my wonderful teenage years I had attempted suicide twice; one time being more serious than the other. Even though that was all dealt with at the time it happened, and hadn't become an issue for over 10 years now, I was sure that this would seem like a good time for the issue to manifest itself again, at least through Mom's eyes. This made me decide to just go home and deal with my sister and her concerns. After all, Mom was probably in the middle of scaring the daylights out of Tammy.

As I pulled into the driveway she must have said, "he's home—gotta go, bye," because I could tell by the expression on Tammy's face that she had been told. She asked me if I was okay, and I could tell that she was at a loss for words. I said, "yeah," but told her I needed some time to myself to work things out. She wanted to know more, but, hell, I didn't know much more than that myself. I did explain to her that she and Shawn (her 2-year-old son) were okay, and that I had to make some phone calls, and I would tell her anything that I could find out.

I carried the groceries through the living room, which now had a dining room table set up in it for tomorrow, and headed into the kitchen. That reminded me of Thanksgiving. How I wished we could just cancel the entire holiday.

When I got to my room, I wanted to just lay back and try to figure out what was going to happen, but I thought I would be better off if I got on the phone right away. I called the number of the first doctor on the referral list. The line was busy. Then I tried the National Hotline. Finally a voice on the other end of the line answered "AIDS Hotline, can I help you?" I remember the man sounded rushed and somewhat tired so I explained to him that I had just gotten a positive test result and. . . . Before I could tell him that I had been sick for the past month he said, "Just because you tested positive doesn't mean you'll ever get sick. Don't have sex and just try to stay healthy. Whatever you do, don't tell anyone. Thanks for calling." Well, that was a big help.

I stopped, took a breath and started calling doctors again. I wondered why, if this disease is so devastating, there were only three names on the list. I got through, but the earliest appointment I could get was a month away. I took it anyway, and thought I would call the other two and cancel this one if I got an earlier appointment somewhere else. Now I'm not a very patient person, but a month? That was ridiculous! I was mad, and also confused. Should I have told them why I was calling, or do I wait and tell the doctor? I didn't know the answer, so I called the other numbers. If I could get an earlier appointment, I wouldn't say anything until I actually saw a doctor. I called the number next to the second name, but it was busy, so I called the third number on my doctor list. I got through and asked to speak directly to the doctor. He had to call me back. I decided that the best thing to do would be to start preparing things for tomorrow's dinner and just wait for him to return my call. I really wanted to cancel the entire dinner. I knew everyone would understand, but then they would also know that something was terribly wrong, and on top of all my problems I didn't want or need to start dealing with their dilemmas. I also wasn't going to allow any illness to take away any of the control I had over my life.

I decided to start working on Thanksgiving dinner by cleaning vegetables while I waited. Every minute I would stop to look at the clock and every minute seemed like 20 until I got that call. It only took about 20 minutes for him to call back, but it seemed like an eternity. This day had seemed like a year-long bad dream that was probably lasting just moments. I remember feeling so tired, so emotionally drained at this point that I could fall asleep. I still hadn't really even started to deal with anything on my own.

The doctor was very nice and patient. I told him about my being ill and my test result. He told me that if I wasn't sick at the moment I really didn't have anything to worry about, but that he would like to see me. There was something in his voice and the way he spoke to me that sounded positive. He connected me to the appointment desk where I got an appointment for 2 weeks from now. Finally. . .a positive note! Two weeks I can deal with. I tried calling to cancel the first appointment I had made, but I got another busy signal and thought the hell with it—I had more important things to worry about. Now, what to do next?

Should I call my friends and my lover? Everybody I've been to bed with in the last 5—no, 7 years! Where does one begin? A lot of these people have moved away and besides, I really don't know that much myself. Is all this stuff ever going to end? Now I'm afraid to stop—afraid to think, because every time I do, things just get more and more confusing, more frightening, and more like I'm going to be dealing with this stuff until I die, which right now doesn't seem that far away.

After calming myself down, I decided to call this phone number they gave me for a place called an AIDS Project. I hated the idea of calling. I guess I stereotype these places to be like social disease clinics, which always make me feel dirty, but I need more information and I need it now. I had met the woman who ran the clinic years ago through a friend, so I thought that would help. I asked a million questions to which they gave me a million answers—"to the best of their ability." This proved to be aggravating—it wasn't what they told me, but the lack of information about the disease that was aggravating. Am I going to die? No one ever wants to answer that and at this point there was no answer. How is it spread? Blood, semen, and again another maybe, saliva. Well, if it's saliva, then what about my family? Well, they didn't think so; no one who treated AIDS patients, including family members, has ever contracted the virus. Then they asked me where I was as far as diagnosis. I didn't understand what that meant and asked them the same question. They explained to me the three categories—antibody positive, ARC, and AIDS. God, this was all so complicated! So they made an appointment for me to come down and see a counselor. They also gave me a number to call for a support group. So I called and made arrangements to get into the support group, which wasn't meeting again until after the holidays. Well, that was okay because I had at least gotten some information and I was going down to see an AIDS counselor in less than a week.

I then decided to read all the pamphlets I had been given at the hospital to see if I could learn anything else. It all seemed so deadly and so glum. While I was reading, my nephew came into my room. Shawn was 2 years old. As he entered the room, the first thing he went for was a glass on my nightstand, looking for something to drink. I jumped back and snapped it out of his hands immediately. As he started to cry, I picked him up and held him so tightly that I was afraid I had hurt him. This, in turn, started me crying. What was happening to me?

I moved into the kitchen and started preparing Thanksgiving dinner so Shawn wouldn't see my pain. I threw myself into the tasks of cooking, baking, and completely preparing the Thanksgiving meal to the point where nothing else could crawl into my brain. Finally, everything was as ready as it could be at this point. It was about 12:30 AM and I was too tired to do anything but go to bed.

I must have been extremely exhausted because it was almost 9 AM when I woke up. I thought about yesterday and fantasized that it was all just a bad dream. The phone started ringing. Of course, it was Mom wondering how I felt. I remember thinking that I hoped this wouldn't become an everyday event. I was sure that for now she needed to hear that I was okay. I told her I had to get back to work and that I would see her around 2:30 PM. From that point on, our telephone conversations would always end with "I love you." Before, if we didn't say it now and then when saying goodbye, it wasn't that important. However, now it was as if saying "I love you" had more priority than the conversation itself.

Little by little, my family started showing up, and what happened was almost funny. First, my younger brother arrived with his wife and two children. Mom must have stressed to them how important my physical health was, because they had brought an "Octagym" with them. They set it up and showed me how it was used. They asked me if I needed any help in the kitchen, completely avoiding the issue of my test results! Finally, my brother asked what happened and I prepared myself for what I would probably be repeating all day long. I told him that this didn't mean that I had AIDS or would ever get it. Also, that he and our family were safe and that it was great that they had brought the machine, so I could keep myself in shape and avoid developing the virus. I tried to make light of the situation, because even though we don't say it to each other, we love each other very much. He never was good at handling or expressing his feelings, but you could feel his concern. Next, my other brother, his wife, and their four children arrived. Along with them came a complete weight-lifting outfit. We had the same conversation I had just completed with my other brother. Then my mom and stepfather arrived. Mom's first reaction was a hug and kisses, which I tried to make light of by explaining how busy I was in the kitchen.

Well, this is the moment I dreaded the most. We were all sitting, ready to eat, and all we had left to do was to say grace. I thought that would probably be the hardest part. I could just picture someone saying something that would make Mom fall apart. My older brother said grace, which he normally does. Probably because he does it best, and this time was no different. It was perfect. Not a word about my test. So dinner went well, except for the tension. Everyone was trying to make small talk. Not one moment of silence was allowed, but the subject of AIDS was never mentioned either. I got up to clear the dishes and bring in the dessert and champagne.

After dessert was served, I poured the champagne and made a toast to the first time we all had a holiday meal at home—and not one fight! Then it happened. Here I had tried to make light of the situation and then Mom stands up. It's all over now, I thought. "There's something you should all know," and Mom went on to tell them what a fight we had ahead of us, and that now would be the time we needed to be a family the most. No one knew what to say. How could they? We didn't know much, but we were pretty scared. After dinner everyone stayed around to help with the cleanup.

The next morning started out very slowly. The mental and physical extremes of the past week had caught up with me. However, I have never been one to just lay around doing nothing. I have always believed that lying around when you don't feel well makes you feel even worse. So, I picked up the materials I had gotten from the hospital to see if I could make some sense out of this disease that I had, or might have, or didn't have. As I read, I got more confused, and the more confused I got, the more intimidated I felt. I never thought of myself as stupid. I've always been able to figure out a way to deal with anything that got in my way, but none of this stuff made any sense—I felt like an idiot.

First, I went through the symptoms: *Purple to red flat or raised blotches that usually are painless.* I checked my body and didn't find anything. *Persistent diarrhea.* I didn't have that. *Rapid, unexplained weight loss.* I didn't have that either; my weight has always been low. Even my nickname in high school was "Stick Man." *Fatigue.* I have that, but nothing extreme or unexplained. *Night sweats, usually extreme and long lasting.* These I had while I was sick, but I got them almost every time I was sick. *High fevers, again long lasting and usually greater than 99 degrees.* These I had while I was sick, but that was normal. *Thrush, a thick coating on the mouth and throat.* I didn't have that one either. *Swollen lymph nodes under armpits, groin area, or neck.* I thought I had some of these, but I wasn't real sure.

Then, after the list of symptoms, they stated that these symptoms were also common to a lot of other illnesses, and that they didn't mean a person had or would ever develop AIDS. Also, the symptoms may mean ARC, which stands for AIDS-related complex. So now that tells me that I may just be a carrier and never get sick or I may develop ARC or I may go on to develop AIDS and die!

I've never liked uncertainty. I've always had control over my life, and now it would all be taken away. I've never been so horrified by anything in my life—not even specifically the disease, but just the idea of not knowing what the future would hold.

Then there was the list of precautions, and some information on how the virus is spread. This only made me feel lethal and dirty. How many people could I have issued a death warrant to? By this time, I wanted to quit. I didn't want to hear any more. I already felt dirty, scared, hurt, confused, and totally out of control. However, I knew I had to learn it all. Knowledge seemed to be the only thing I could use as a defense at this time. So I finished reading everything, but still didn't learn much.

I decided to try and figure out how I could have been exposed to the virus, which would make it a little easier to decide how far back into my past I would have to go to inform everyone who needed to be concerned. The past year was easy. I have had a monogamous relationship. Then it dawned on me that his previous lover was a male prostitute, but that didn't allow much of an incubation period. Then there was George who had died in September, which again didn't allow much of an incubation period.

Wait a minute, this is ridiculous, I thought. I could never be sure, and besides it wasn't going to prove anything anyway. If I was going to tell anyone, it would eventually travel to the public anyway. This would probably stop me from ever going out again. I wouldn't want to deal with the gossip, and I never could deal with pity. Besides, maybe I wouldn't even get served with all the fears and misconceptions people have about this disease. There were also a lot of good things that could come out of going public. The word might get to people that I had no way of getting in touch with, and maybe with all the people I knew in the gay community, just maybe they would get the message that AIDS was hitting home and they would start taking the necessary precautions to save their lives. I wasn't sure what to do.

I decided to start by telling Paul, a long-time friend of mine. I didn't want him to find out through the grapevine. Once on the phone, we talked about how we spent our Thanksgivings. Forgetting why I called, I felt contented. As the conversation was coming to an end, I remembered why I called, and instantly these feelings changed to fear and pain.

Once off the phone, I was in tears. I felt so guilty and so helpless. Everything was being taken away from me. The worst part was that I had no control, and I couldn't stop it from destroying anyone else either. It wasn't bad enough that this was happening to me, but that I had inflicted this on an undetermined number of others.

The only thing I could do to stop myself from falling apart was to concentrate on something totally different. I decided to find a spot for all of the exercise equipment. I set everything up and read every instruction manual. Doing this took my mind off everything else.

About an hour later, the phone rang. It was Mike, my friend from high school. I really wasn't in the mood for company, I was emotionally exhausted, but to keep up my strong front I invited him over. I thought about all the questions he would have, and how tired I was getting of answering them, but there really wasn't anything that could change that. I jumped in the shower, thinking that might help to make me feel better, and it did seem to help. I felt clean and ready to start with my strong exterior again.

When Mike walked in, he could hardly believe the way my room looked with all the exercise equipment in it. We joked about it for a moment, but I could tell what was ahead. Sure enough, the questions came: How was I? What did the hospital say? Was it very contagious? *Was he safe?* We covered it all one more time. The only problem was that there weren't enough answers. Even though I told him all I could, he was still justifiably scared.

Today being Saturday, I decided I would go out to some of the bars that I used to go to and start to try and contact people. I wasn't real fond of doing it this way, but I really didn't know how else to find some of these people. Before I went out, I gave Paul a call. One more time, I had to tell the story. After telling him, I told him that I would stop at the bar where he worked and talk to him in person. When I got to the bar, an uneasy feeling came over me, as if people were staring at me. At first I thought it was just my imagination, but the bartender handed me a drink and apologized to me. Then the bar manager offered his condolences. At first I was mad and I wanted to go to the back bar where Paul was working and wring his neck. He must have seen me come in from the window, because by the time I got back to him he was in tears. I really couldn't start yelling at him. He explained to me that he only told the people he thought I would want to know. I couldn't argue with him because I hadn't told him to keep it a secret. So instead, I comforted him the best I could and we had a couple drinks together. Then the bar started getting busy, so I decided to start hitting some other places. The first person I ran into was real hard to tell and I thought it would get easier, but it didn't. By the end of the evening, I was exhausted. I felt like I had destroyed so many people's evenings, so many people's lives. One more time, I would cry myself to sleep.

The next morning, another friend of mine phoned and his first response wasn't "hello" but "Hi, is it true?" Jim and I had been the best of friends until I moved to the country. We were still close, but had gone off in our own directions. So one more time I had to go through a question and answer period that I was starting to refer to as AIDS 101. After that call, I was a mess. I was falling apart emotionally, and finally admitted to myself that I needed help. I pulled myself together and gave the AIDS Project a call. They were very friendly and set up an appointment for me to come down and talk to someone. When I got off the phone, a part of me was disappointed that I couldn't handle this on my own, but another part of me knew I was becoming self-destructive.

Two Years Later

Aids and I have shared about 2 years together. In this time, I've gone through a lot of changes in my life. My entire outlook on life has drastically changed. I learned to deal with AIDS as a part of my life, and have gone through dying of AIDS to living with AIDS.

AIDS implies more than an illness. It allows itself to manifest into a number of ugly controversies. It isn't bad enough that as an illness it destroys a person in any way it chooses, that people become ill and die, that there are times it seems to play games. In my case, AIDS has chosen to play it's evil games. One minute I'm hospitalized with an illness that anyone could slough off, but not an AIDS patient. It slowly wears you down until paranoia of death sets in. Then, you win that fight and the virus seems to leave you alone for a time, as if to allow you to build your strength up again to the point where it causes mind games. You feel healthy, sometimes healthy enough to believe you don't even have AIDS. Then, when you least expect it, BANG! It attacks again. As if the illnesses AIDS brings aren't enough, the virus likes to hide, to make things as hard as possible for the medical profession, to create exorbitant hospital bills that can cause financial disaster. Along with leaving me ill on and off, and financially in ruin, it wasn't about to stop until death became a wish. Peace and serenity seemed impossible until I admitted I had lost and allowed AIDS to take it's toll. And this is still not enough. AIDS doesn't just attack me, but everyone in my life. Every hospitalization would put a scare into my family and friends. The society that surrounded me would now have to deal with its own fears. Fears that would be distorted by the media. Bigoted groups, calling themselves Christians, said we were all damned to die as a punishment from God.

I decided from an early point in my illness that I couldn't allow these attitudes to affect me. I truly believe that God is on my side, allowing me the privilege of knowing what my future may hold in store, allowing me to go from shutting others out of my life to giving me the closest, most loving relationships that anyone could ever conceive. And through His mercy, surrounding me with all of this love, I have developed strength. The strength to go on fighting and to live my life as fully as possible. The strength to try and help others through their struggles, and the strength to help educate others, so that they may help, and bestow a little love and compassion to help give others the strength to go on fighting. This is a fight I intend to win, as I feel I have already.

I started out confused and afraid. Two years later I no longer feel either of these. Instead, I feel loved and optimistic for the future. Not that there aren't any more problems or fears, but that at least AIDS has been put in it's place in my life. It's an illness and just that.

I'll conquer each problem as it arises with a positive outlook for the future, and if my life should end, I'll be at peace knowing I did my best. I hope everyone in my life who played a major part in helping me find strengths I never even knew I had will know too.

Todd Butler died at home with his mother and his partner, Michael, on August 21, 1988. What follows is Michael's story of the time he had with Todd.

MICHAEL'S STORY

In the summer of 1986, I was working at a local AIDS Service Organization. In mid-August, we had a small reception to announce the opening of our library. I saw Todd for the first time at that party. It was an appropriate setting—Todd loved to party, have fun, be active and alive. I am less comfortable in that setting. He possessed many qualities I wish I had. He was outgoing—at times, outrageous—never afraid to say what he felt and never afraid of what others might think. Todd was at ease in almost any setting. He talked easily with new people. He liked to entertain. I understood all of this over time, but in that moment when I first saw him, I was simply drawn to him. I will never forget how he looked that night. When he smiled, his eyes actually sparkled.

A few weeks later, I went to another party—this one was to celebrate Todd's 30th birthday. In the time between parties, I learned that Todd had AIDS. I went to the party in part because I felt someone from our agency should be there. After all, Todd had sent a blanket invitation to the staff and volunteers. (I learned later that he was hoping I would attend.) I didn't relish going to a party alone, but I wanted to see Todd, to get to know him. It was a large party, and we spoke briefly several times during the evening. But before I left the party, I looked for Todd in the crowd so that I could say goodnight to him. When I found him, we hugged, and then I kissed him. I remember thinking, you've just kissed a person with AIDS, and just as quickly thinking—so what? Through reading at work, I knew that a simple kiss on the lips posed no risk of infection. Reading is one thing, doing is another. For me, with that first kiss came the realization that a relationship with Todd was not precluded by AIDS.

Over the next few weeks, Todd and I met by chance several times, then we began to plan the meetings. Our first attempt at having sex didn't work out. Todd feared that somehow, despite precautions, I could become infected. I had been tested before I met Todd and was HIV negative. I had spent a lot of time learning about and teaching others about safer sex, and I wanted to put what I had learned into action. My fear that I would expose Todd to a cold or flu was far greater than my fear of becoming infected with HIV. So that night, instead of having sex, we lay in bed together, cuddling and talking. Todd felt that maybe we should stop ourselves from going any farther with the relationship. He felt he could only hurt me—physically, by possibly infecting me and emotionally, by dying.

Todd's emotional impact on me was so strong that I knew his death would affect me even if I never saw him again. I wanted to see him and make the best of whatever time we had left. We decided to keep seeing each other.

Those early days of our relationship were happy. Todd was feeling well and we were learning new things about each other. Todd volunteered time at my agency, so 2 or 3 days a week we would go to work and come home together. I had accepted from the start that the most likely end of our relationship would be Todd's death. At the time, though, Todd was healthy, we were happy, and I didn't dwell on his having AIDS or his possible death. Too soon, though, things would change.

A few days before Halloween, Todd had a biopsy done on some inflamed tissue in his lower left leg. That Friday night, our agency was sponsoring a concert and costume party fund-raiser. We spent the day buying pumpkins, cornstalks, and streamers to decorate for the party. In the afternoon, Todd got a phone call from the doctor's office—the biopsy results were back. Todd wanted to go to his doctor alone, so I waited at the office. When he returned he said the tests indicated early Kaposi's sarcoma. I think we were both numbed by the news and trying hard to be brave for each other. I noticed that he had some gauze wrapped around his hand. When I asked about it he said that it was just a scrape, nothing really. Later he told me he'd punched a wall in a bathroom at the hospital.

Todd wanted some time away from me that afternoon. He needed some time to digest the news. He left for a couple of hours. I talked with Susan, my boss, while he was gone. She had known Todd for a few years. Todd said I could tell her about the Kaposi's sarcoma. We hugged and cried, and managed to put on brave faces by the time Todd returned. I knew Todd had AIDS, but I somehow thought we would have a year or so before anything really serious happened, and I just didn't think about his diagnosis that often. In retrospect, the Kaposi's sarcoma didn't cause too many problems for Todd. He didn't develop more lesions until very near the end of his life. But at that time, I felt like I had been slapped across the face unexpectedly. AIDS was reminding me that it was there, and that I couldn't ignore it.

We went to the Halloween party that night anyway. On the way, we stopped at a bar for a drink because Todd wanted to tell me something. I remember being afraid that he was going to suggest we break up before things got too rough. Instead, he gave me a ring he always wore and told me he loved me. He said it was an early birthday present in case anything happened before then. What follows are the occasional journal entries I made during my relationship with Todd.

October 21, 1986

Where the hell have I been? Nothing written in here since July— didn't anything happen? Last night we (Todd, Lynn, Dawn, and I) were at Dawn's apartment. She mentioned writing in her journal. I need to write, and have needed to for many weeks now, especially about everything happening with Todd. He called this morning before I left for school. When he said he wasn't good, I was instantly afraid he was getting sick. I feel guilty because I'm fighting off a cold and still staying close to him. I don't know what I would do if he got sick because of me. I need to talk to him about this. Todd said last night that maybe we should call it quits before we get too involved, but I think it's too late. At this point, I already feel strongly enough about him that I'll be devastated when he dies, even if I don't see him again. I'm not afraid of getting AIDS from him—sometimes I think I already have it—and sometimes I wish I did have it. I'm not afraid to die. What scares me is that I might speed Todd's death by seeing him. I have a lot to say to Todd. I think he is feeling the same way. Right now I long to see him and hold him and talk to him, but I'm afraid when

I do see him, I'll clam up. Sometimes so much love swells up in me, but when I'm near him I can't show it. Does this relate to Martin? I loved him so much and only got hurt for it. Am I still afraid of being hurt again? Paralyzed by fear?

Todd and I have to talk about relationships. We seem to have reached the point where we take the next set of risks—beyond just saying we care for each other or want to see each other. Do I really give myself to him—my whole heart—like I think I did with Martin? And in his case, am I worth dying for? Seeing me could shorten his life. Could seeing me make his life longer, if I make him happy? We really have gotten into a difficult situation.

October 27, 1986

I love Todd more each day. Today I went to Mary's father's funeral with him. He is so dear to me. I don't want the day to come when I have to attend Todd's funeral. I realize how important it is for me to tell him how much I care for him. I love him.

June 27, 1987

I haven't written in this notebook for 8 months. So much has happened. I will take this to work with me, and write some there. Right now I'm too dizzy from my sleeping pill to write—till tomorrow then.

January 5, 1988

So much for writing tomorrow. No more sleeping pills. I wish I had one. I'm afraid. Todd is sick, feverish, sweating, not eating. Bernice, his mother, called me at home. I'm here because it's so cold—minus 10 degrees this morning—and my car wouldn't start. I want to be there with Todd. I want to hold him, keep him warm with my body. Bernice usually overreacts, so I hope he isn't as bad as she made it sound. He wants to die. I'm afraid. I don't want him to die, and I don't want it to happen tonight, not when I'm not there. Please God keep him warm, keep him alive at least until I'm with him. I love him. I'm going to sleep now. I'm afraid my whole life will be different tomorrow. I don't want that—I'm not ready yet. But he said he thought it would be the second week of January. Please God, not yet.

January 6, 1988

Todd is alive! I talked to him twice. The first time he sounded better. The second time, he was pissed, in the Joan Crawford mode, so I'm at home. It was -10 degrees again today, I'm depressed by the cold and my non-functional $198.15-per-month car. Tomorrow it will be towed to the dealer. The video we watched at work darkened my mood. It was the march on Washington! Scenes of the Names Project Quilt had me torn up emotionally. AIDS is so cruel. I find myself crying for people I don't even know and over losses that aren't even mine. My heart aches for Todd at those times. I miss him so—and he isn't even gone yet. Please God, send a cure soon. I finished reading *The Lost Language of Cranes*—excellent! But, as with all good books, I feel empty now that it's done. I want it to go on. Fortunately, I still have half of the *Accidental Tourist*. Enough for now. Take care of yourself, Michael!

January 11, 1988

It's late, I'm home. I read some of Todd's diaries. I feel like a kid who's done something wrong, but he said I could look at them. Pretty normal stuff. It's always nice when my name is mentioned. This weekend we went to Madison, on Friday we delivered grants to the Department of Health, and on Saturday we stayed at the Embassy Suites. Todd permed my hair and his mom's. Hers looks really nice. Todd and I made love that night—as he said, for the first time in 1988. I love him. Sunday he was worn out. We went to bed around 7 PM. He fell asleep instantly. I watched TV and read Lawrence Sander's *The Third Deadly Sin*. Todd cuddled up to me all evening. That's about the only nice thing about his being sick. He has some new purple spots and cytomegalovirus (CMV) in his eyes. I'm afraid the end is near. I hope not. I love him. It's midnight—time for bed.

I wish I'd written more. AIDS is horrible. I don't want to say that there is anything good about it, yet it has brought many things to me. AIDS has given me challenging work, and the feeling that I am doing something important, something that matters. If it weren't for my involvement in the fight against AIDS, I might never have met Todd Butler.

Todd wanted to do something important, too. He wanted to show people what it was like to live with AIDS. He wanted to touch people's lives, and change ignorance and fear into understanding. To do this, he began speaking publicly about his illness. He appeared on television and radio, and he did a series of newspaper interviews. He also wrote.

Todd intended to write a book about his experience with AIDS. He wrote five chapters. He had been diagnosed with full-blown AIDS about a year before we met. The chapters he wrote cover much of that year. Some of the chapters are difficult for me to read. He talks about another lover. I long to read what he would have written about me. Still, I treasure the chapters I have. Todd put his feelings—especially his fears—on paper, with a sense of openness and honesty that was difficult for him to express in person.

Todd stopped writing late in 1987. Only he knew the true reasons why. I know he wanted to tell his whole story, and I suspect he reached a point where it would be difficult to continue honestly without hurting some people he loved very much. Todd died leaving his book unfinished.

I encourage anyone whose life has been touched by AIDS or HIV infection to write. From someone with AIDS, writing can be a priceless gift for loved ones. I am grateful for the writing Todd left in my care. It has given me a better idea of what he went through before we met, as well as greater understanding of Todd and our relationship. For anyone with AIDS or HIV infection, or for people like myself who are close to someone with AIDS or HIV, writing can be a healing process. During my time with Todd, I only occasionally wrote in my journal. I regret that I didn't write more. Looking back at what we both wrote, and thinking about my life with Todd while writing this, has really helped me to lay some painful memories to rest. It has also brought back some happy memories that had been clouded by thoughts of illness and death.

12

Living Under the Sword

Tony Rizzolo

My name is Tony and I'm a recovering addict. I tell you I'm a recovering addict because it gives you an idea of how I caught this virus, but how I caught it isn't really important, it's how I'm handling it now that's important.

You see, this virus is probably the best thing that has ever happened to me. When I tell people this, they look at me like I'm still on drugs. They don't understand what I've been through. They don't understand the lessons that this virus has taught me. For 20 years I complained that life wasn't worth it, that it stunk. And you know what the virus taught me? It taught me what life was all about. Before, I was always walking into hospitals and Alcoholics Anonymous meetings asking everyone else for the answers. Then the virus blinded me and I found all the answers I needed right inside. When I came down with a skin problem, being blind was an advantage because I didn't have to see what my skin problem looked like. And the skin problem taught me patience, that this too shall pass, and it did. Then I picked up a second virus. I mean, the doctors had a hospital room ready for me. They said it was going to start attacking my nervous system. I got so frustrated that I looked at the spot where the virus came in and I said, "You heard that, well don't even try it because you ain't staying." I actually talked to the virus, I wrote down my visualizations, I attacked the little sucker with everything possible—exercise, diet, positive thinking, and humor. I came at it from all sides. That virus is probably dizzy. See, cause if I can't win um I'll spin um. And today I've got that little sucker running in circles. It's attacked me in just about every spot possible. But I keep managing to cut out of this.

The key word in my vocabulary today is resiliency. It's the ability to keep bouncing back no matter how many times you get knocked down. And I've been knocked down a lot in the past 18 months. It's been one problem after the other—from pneumonia to blindness to skin problems to the second virus to going to the funerals of friends I

---

lost to AIDS, and friends and relatives I lost to cancer—it's either one or the other. But as long as I can keep the focus on myself, everything is going to be okay.

Today I'm a winner because today I wake up and I deal with life on life's terms. I don't have to drug myself to get through the day. And that's a miracle, because if you knew my MO—I mean, I got high on the bad days, then I got high on the good days because I thought they should be bad. Hey, I didn't need an excuse to get high. It's unbelievable that I asked my higher power to give me just one weapon to fight the disease of addiction. Just one. And the one time he answers me, look what he gives me, a virus. Do you know that old saying—be careful what you ask for, you just might get it? Boy did I get it. But he know a little more than me, he knew exactly what I needed. Because for 20 years I couldn't stay straight out there. Now all of a sudden I've got this virus and I went blind and found all the answers I needed. I know how to stay straight today. You see, I can't affect one disease without hitting the other. If I thought I was going to die of AIDS, I'd go out and get high. But if I went out and got high, I probably would die of AIDS. If I fall to one disease I fall to the other. And if I'm beating one I'm automatically beating the other one. It's strange how for 20 years I didn't have any of these answers.

Someone once asked me how I finally got the message and I thought of this little story.

I saw an alcoholic passing by an open window and the alcoholic looked in and saw a woman praying to God saying, "please just give me one loaf of bread, just one, I'm hungry." Now the alcoholic outside, he's laughing, "look at this maniac praying to someone she can't even see. I'm going to teach her a lesson." So he goes to the corner grocery store, buys a loaf of bread, comes back and throws it in the window. The woman picks up the loaf of bread and says "Thank you, God." Now the alcoholic is mad so he sticks his head in the window and says "Miss, I gave you that loaf of bread." So the woman says "No, that came from a higher power." The guy says, "No, miss, I gave it to you." And the woman turns around and says, "No, that came from a higher power." So the guy says, "Listen ma'am, I spent two bucks on that loaf of bread, it came from me," and the woman turns around and says, "Let me tell you something sucker, that loaf of bread came from a higher power. He just had to get the devil to deliver it." This explains exactly what I have been through.

For 20 years my higher power has been tapping me on the shoulder saying, "Hey, son, you're doing the wrong thing." And I ignored him. But when the virus delivered the message, I sat up and listened. It's amazing to see how thick-headed I was and how far I've come. But everyone needs help in his own way. I'm exactly where I'm supposed to be today. A lot of times I claim that my life isn't where I'd like it to be. But thank God it's not where it was. I've just got to be grateful that I'm exactly where I am today.

Today I go out and I talk to students. I've talked to teachers. I've been invited out to StonyBrook twice, to Mary Immaculate Hospital. I just got through with a presentation at a college of physicians and surgeons. Would you believe this, people paying me $200. to see and hear what me and some other people have to say! I mean, there was a time when people would pay me so that I wouldn't open my mouth. I was always confusing the hell out of everyone. But today, thanks to this virus, I have a higher quality of life. For 20 years I was like the walking dead. Now that I've picked up this virus new channels are open to me. Would you believe that I just got back from California a couple of days ago, and some people actually invited me over to their house? When I was active, no one ever invited me over, if they made that mistake, they didn't make another by giving me the right address. What's happening to me today is a miracle—when I was leaving they actually asked me to come back. That's one thing people never said to me. And like I said, I owe a lot to this virus. But it's only because I made it through the pain that I've had these good days to enjoy. Sometimes you have to go through the storm before you can get to the sunshine. And sometimes the only thing in that storm is one ray of sunshine to hang on to. And the only thing positive about it is that I'm dealing with the storm without picking up a drink or a drug. But you know what? When the sun comes out in my backyard it comes out a little brighter because I've made it through the storm. Now I try to get this message across to other people. Because there are people out there who, when they find out they have the virus, go out and get high, and when they go out and get high the virus goes berserk. Putting drugs in front of the virus is like putting blood in front of a shark. Once you do that, there's no turning back.

Hopefully there are people out there who will listen to my message. Because when you want to attack the disease of AIDS you have to attack it from all sides. You can't just talk to gays. The gays listen, but with addicts, their priorities are so screwed up, that it's hard to get them under the same roof. Addicts spend all their energy every day just getting what they need, from the time they get up in the morning and get their money together, to finding the right connection, to getting there without getting busted, then getting back without getting beat, and needing to find a place to do it in. I'm tired just thinking about all the running around I did. If we could take 10% of that energy and attack the virus with it, what a dent we'd make! It's like breaking that one link in the chain, the link that goes from the addict to the girl he's going with, to the baby they have who has AIDS. Break that one link, and the baby would never wind up with it. Somewhere along the line we have to find a way to get through to the addicts. What I'm talking to you about isn't just addiction or AIDS, its about life under the sword. And for me, it's life under two swords. Because its only through the second sword that I found out how to deal with the first. Hopefully, not everyone needs to get the message the way I got it. I'm the type that has to keep putting his hand over the match to find out it still burns. I can't learn from someone else's experience. Hopefully not everyone is as thick as I am. And maybe whoever is reading this will get something out of it. I don't know, there's so much more I could say to you. I hope this message gets through and maybe if things work out right I'll be able to come and give you this message in person. Thanks. I want to finish with one last comment. I wouldn't take my worst day with the virus for my best day with the drugs and alcohol because if I die tomorrow I will die a winner because I fought today. For the first time in my life I'm no longer part of the problem but just for today I'm a good part of the solution.

13

Sustaining Hope and Care in the Face of AIDS

Rev. Jennifer M. Phillips, PhD

"I don't know how you can do that work! Don't you find it depressing?" I suspect that every AIDS caregiver has heard this again and again from friends and family, from passing acquaintances and strangers, even from patients. If your answer to this question is "yes", you have probably left AIDS caregiving, or will soon be leaving the field, and appropriately so, for your own well-being. If you are new to the field, I invite you to let the question resonate within you, to be asked again as time goes by. For those of us who for some time have been working with, loving, and giving care to people with AIDS-related illness and their families one might ask, how is it that we sustain our caring long-term without depression and despair? Each of us has our own answers. The larger community needs to hear these answers in order to manage its own fear and depression, now, and increasingly in the years ahead. In this chapter I will share some of my own reflections on and experiences in sustaining hope and care in the face of AIDS, as well as some of the thoughts and methods reported to me by my colleagues in nursing, social work, medicine, and pastoral care.

REASONS FOR DESPAIR

At the time of this writing, reported cases of AIDS in the U.S. have passed the 50,000 mark, and that figure is merely the tip of the iceberg of worldwide disease and infection that falls short of the AIDS diagnosis. Mortality among those diagnosed with AIDS is over 50%. The odds on progression from HIV asymptomatic infection to disease seem greater with every new report of research findings. The disease is spreading outward from the pockets of the population where it first emerged, without respect to color, age, gender, or sexual orientation. Top scientists concur that the likelihood of an effective vaccine or curative treatment is slim this side of the turn of the century. American educational efforts remain bogged down in arguments over morality, language, and political jurisdiction, despite the evidence that education is the only effective means of prevention we now possess. Community agencies, volunteer organizations, and even government and private institutions providing AIDS services see caseloads rising, and the diversity of needs increasing. And in many cases, workers are growing weary as the numbers of the dear and remembered dead move from the dozens to the hundreds. These are some of the many factors that produce discouragement and exhaustion in the AIDS care network.

For many caregivers, as for patients, everyday reality resembles living in a time of war. A patient named David, a gay man in his early twenties, said to me, "I wasn't surprised when the doctors gave me my diagnosis. Over 30 of my friends have already been diagnosed and a lot of them are dead. Why should I be exempt?" Another gay man with AIDS, when I told him of the death of a mutual friend said "I feel as though I'm the last one left alive in my generation." Unlike wartime, however, with AIDS there is no outside enemy to hate (though some focus their anger on the government), there is only the virus within: invisible, minute, intimate, and deadly. Since AIDS has not been accepted by the society as a commonly shared tragedy, there is none of the rallying spirit of a nation at war. Instead, there is isolation, the fragmenting of infected groups from the general population, scapegoating, and denial. For caregivers and patients, in the gay community in particular, death is experienced not only as individual, but also as the death of a whole culture at the point it was beginning to be recognized and to blossom. The need for communal grieving is great.

Andy, a member of a people with AIDS (PWA) group, confided to me, "I sometimes feel guilty just walking into my PWA group. If I am feeling up and good, it's not okay because so many people are not doing well. If I feel tired and sad and want to cry or just give up, it's not okay to show that because you're supposed to keep a good positive attitude and not bring people down." At times, the same dynamic operates in the helping network, where the constant loss causes grief that's likely to be suppressed in the urgency of moving on to meet the next need, thus a chronic depression sets in which makes moments of celebration impossible. The community neither mourns nor celebrates wholeheartedly, but simply tries to keep moving on as fast as possible. The energy caregivers need for their work tends to diminish when their emotions are ignored or suppressed. In popular jargon, this phenomenon has been labeled "burnout," which I believe is largely the effect of grieving left undone.

BALANCE OF VISION

It is a universal truth that if one stares at the sun too long, one may go blind. There may be a similar truth about death: that one cannot stare death in the face for too long without looking away, or one will lose the ability to see anything else.

As a pastor to hospitalized PWAs I make my initial visit, perhaps becoming engrossed in the person's story, feelings, and whatever distinguishes that individual as being unique and engaging. A few hours later as I review the visit mentally, it strikes me that this is indeed a person with AIDS who will likely die within 2 years, if not in the next few weeks or days. Sadness accompanies the thought, and needs a little time to be recognized and felt. Then my attention shifts again to whatever the ongoing needs may be as expressed by the person and their loved ones. Death is still in the picture, but moves from the center of the frame to a corner of the larger perspective of the life now being lived. It seems helpful to me to observe this inner shift with some intentionality. One metaphor I find eloquent is that of a pond. Sitting beside the water, I am drawn to the sparkle of the surface as the wind ripples it. When it stills, the sun and clouds and blueness of the sky are reflected in a delightful brilliance. Then the eye is drawn by a darkness at the margin, and pulled down into the depths where mouldering leaves lie and grey stones and rotting sticks litter the bottom in a landscape of decay. Both views are real, and are available to the eye at any moment; yet they have a very different feeling tone, the one vibrant with light and color, the other gloomy and repelling. It is possible to look at our experience of working with the dying in a similar way: seeing the courage and tenacity of the processes of life and even the hopeful images of afterlife, or confronting the dissolution of body and sometimes of mind in the process of dying and the sadness of the space the dead leave behind in us. It is a spiritual discipline worth cultivating to be able to look upon both realities and move between them fluidly; to bear in mind the one while experiencing the other, and not to get stuck in either one.

People with AIDS are themselves moving between the two poles, not experiencing stages of dying, but fluctuating between moments of hope and despair, of fighting and surrendering, of anger and healing, of faith and fear. Insofar as we can travel beside them keeping pace, we are likely to be of help.

In the poetic prayer of the Judeo-Christian tradition in the Psalms, I hear the echo of the caregiver's perspective, seeing the darkness:

> For my soul is full of troubles,
> and my life draws near to Sheol.
> I am reckoned among those who go down to the pit.
> I am one who has no strength,
> like one lost among the dead . . .
>
> *(Psalm 88)*

and being drawn back to the light:

> For Thou hast delivered my soul from death,
> my eyes from tears, my feet from stumbling;
> I walk before the Lord in the land of the living.
> I kept my faith, even when I said,
> "I am greatly afflicted" . . .
> Precious in the eyes of the Lord
> is the death of his saints.
>
> *(Psalm 116)*

Maintaining a balanced vision is one way of sustaining hope and care. To do this effectively, we need a community to say to each of us when we are feeling lost among the dead, "there is life here also."

BEFRIENDING OUR MORTALITY

Many AIDS patients are 25 to 40 years old. A majority of AIDS caregivers are also 25 to 40 years old. In this respect, when we look at our patients we may easily see ourselves. This makes the temptation to magnify the differences, (maybe a homosexual orientation, or a needle-using habit, or even an equatorial foreign culture) considerable. When we watch their dying we encounter our own inevitable mortality. When we hear their grieving or anger, it likely touches our own. At times this is enough to make the calmest among us turn and run: to humor, to denial, to some other patient room, to some other line of work, or whatever. Sometimes our patients need to escape too, and we can do it constructively together. Sometimes there is no place for them to hide even for a moment, and they need us to stay present and tolerate the pain with them.

In medieval times, when life, by comparison to our own modern American life, was "nasty, brutish, and short," there were exercises designed to help faithful souls prepare for their own deaths. Many of these disciplines, which sprang up in, but were not confined to monastic communities, involve preparing to stand before the judgment seat of an exacting deity. These may be less useful for the modern or secular person. More useful are suggestions about guided imagery and meditation, in which one takes stock of life to see whether, if one were to die today, relationships and business and one's spiritual state are where one would wish them to be. The attitude toward living created by the regular use of meditation upon one's dying is one of detachment (in the sense of knowing that all possessions and activities are ephemeral), and of living in the present, with a minimum of unfinished business, unhealed wounds given or received, and unspoken *words* of importance. As the spiritual classic *The Imitation of Christ* puts it, "Thou oughtest in every deed and thought so to order thyself as if thou wert to die this day."

Another step toward befriending our mortality may be the planning of our funeral and making of a will. I make a will each birthday as a spiritual exercise; as for my funeral, after many revisions it contains so many hymns that I "can't live without" that my friends are sure to be heartily sorry that I have died by the time they get through it (if they don't have the good sense to ignore it and do their own thing!). Imagining our deathbed scene, dying experience, and funeral may also be a route to acquaintance with death. As we come to know ourselves as living, but also dying persons, death is transformed from the Grim Reaper, the enemy, to the Gentle Sister Death of St. Francis of Assisi's understanding.

Making peace with the deaths of others requires rituals of mourning; I encourage you to develop your own. Mine range from regular attendance at the Eucharist where I am fed and renewed in both the Good Friday and the Easter Sunday experience of my faith, to sending a bereaved family a note on the 6-month, 1- and 2-year anniversaries of a patient's death, to daily immersion in the womb of my bathtub, to keeping a calendar on which I record the deaths of special people I have known, to attending an occasional funeral service, keeping a prayer list for those who have died, and telling their stories where they need to be heard; and I do miles and miles of walking. It is important to observe a death soon after it occurs by a "time out" from the busy routine of the day, even if all you can take is five minutes; find a place apart in which to be quiet, remember and feel, in order to honor the dead one and yourself and the mystery of the journey.

RESPONSIBILITY AND CONTROL

Next to the failure to do ongoing, daily grief work, one of the greatest contributors to caregivers' exhaustion and depression is close identification with the plight of patients and their families, which tends to generate a powerful need to try to bring relief and change for both them and us. One of the subtle manifestations of this dynamic among the most sensitive and well-meaning of helpers can be the fixation on an image of "the good death." A generation of us have grown up with Elisabeth Kübler-Ross's observations on dying, and those of us in hospital work may have actually experienced the peacefulness of the patient who, having settled all her or his affairs, gathers the family round the bedside, tells them that they are loved, says a prayer, and surrenders quietly to death. Now acceptance of death is not a bad thing for those who have had the time to prepare for and befriend their dying and who are ready to release and be released by their families. For others, it seems uniquely appropriate that they die as they have lived, full of fire and passion, in the middle of their plans and dreams, and angry about going. I've sat with a young man with small children, a deep faith, but a powerful love of his life, who through the last hours shouted "I don't want to die! I don't want to die!" It was agonizing for his nurses to see and hear; they felt that they had failed to help him get ready in some way; yet it was in perfect harmony with who he was. Love asks of us that we let go of our need to have others live or die as we wish they would.

Our role is often simply to be witnesses of others' life and death. I feel this strongly when I have the occasion to sit with a dying person whom I have never known while conscious. I've never met the family or friends, know nothing about what they did or where they came from, never exchanged a word with that person; yet I am a witness to the mystery of their being and their leaving life.

Each person's journey is his own. We may be invited to enter in for a while as a companion and to feel with them, but their sorrows are not ours; the sadness we feel, or the anger, or other emotion is our own. We are responsible for knowing the difference. That clarity of boundaries allows the loving, letting go, moving in and out in relationship and reinvesting in the next relationship which caregiving requires, whether we are chaplains, nurses, social workers, volunteers, doctors, or therapists, kin, or simply friends.

To sustain care, we need to know the limits of our responsibility. We offer the best we have; we are not responsible for the outcome . . . not even if we are physicians! So much of loving those who have AIDS involves simply tolerating our own helplessness: sitting with it, often beside a patient and family who also feel helpless, and not avoiding or trying to disguise it with busyness, unneeded assistance, or enforced cheer.

Medicine in North America has moved in the direction of full disclosure and truth-telling to patients. Informed consent is a watchword in the hospital. Professionals are on the lookout for denial in patients, which may be perceived as the patients' failure to take responsibility for their own truth. Battering those who are seen as in denial with repetitions of the truth is neither effective nor kind.

> "For those with AIDS, especially the newly diagnosed, denial is often a way of managing the terror, a way of coping, of meeting the changes little by little, at one's own pace. What looks like denial from the outside-in may, from the inside-out, allow the space to exert control, to harness the will and resources for survival."
> (Steve Peskind, Further Note on Living with AIDS,
> *Buddhist AIDS Project Newsletter* December 1987)

Knowing the difference between denial, which prevents a patient from seeking their own well-being, and the need to turn the eyes away from staring at the sun too long has much to do with being able to contain one's own helplessness.

In balance, truth-telling is important in relation to the same dynamic. A young man being successfully treated for his pneumocystis pneumonia, but steadily losing weight until he had reached 92 pounds, said to me, "The doctors just came in and said, 'you're doing well.' My nurses keep telling me I'm looking better, I'm breathing better. Can't anyone see that I'm disappearing? I'm disappearing and no one seems to notice." My suspicion is that it is not that John's caregivers did not notice that he was wasting away, but that because they felt helpless to change that process, they were consciously or unconsciously choosing not to notice. When I confirmed that I could see the change in him, John decided that the truth he was experiencing was indeed accurate and he brought the subject up with his doctors and asked about supplemental nutrition, which was then provided for him. It can be hard for a person to know his own truth if they hear untruth from those around them.

We cannot control the processes of dying beyond altering the environment in which they are occurring and reframing the meaning which they have for us. We are merely midwives for the journeys of others; we will sustain our caring better if we are content with that role and if we can trust that in some way there are arms to catch each of us when we slide out of this world into the next, just as there were arms to catch us as we emerged into this world.

BALANCE OF ACTIVITY

Care of others requires good care of self. Nurses in particular among caregivers seem to be developing methods of self-care and describing them in their professional literature. Use of meditation and the relaxation response, along with progressive muscle relaxation, positive affirmations, and guided imagery, is increasing both for pain and stress management with patients and for stress management for staff. We are all more aware of the value of play; both of the institutions with which I am affiliated hired humorists to do staff programs in the last year. The dark humor of emergency caregivers is famous, or infamous, thanks to films and television programs like *MASH* and *St. Elsewhere* and *Hill Street Blues*. The distorting mirror of such humor can be helpful for coping with an intolerable reality as long as it does not occur at the expense of a more vulnerable person. In fact, our patients may be our teachers in this. One patient in his terminal admission was asked by the psychiatrist, "How bad do you think things are?" to which he answered, "Well, I don't buy any green bananas!"

One of the balancing activities I find most useful in AIDS ministry is being a prevention educator. Helping people become informed and move beyond their fear, teaching what they need to know to remain healthy, and putting AIDS in the context of a larger picture of human sexuality that is predominately joyful and life-giving offsets some of the helplessness and loss I feel in working with the sick.

Cooking a meal, digging a garden, making love to a partner, or being musically or artistically creative are all life-affirming ways to achieve balance. If your work does not allow time and energy for such things, you are doing too much work. If you work daily with the physical misery of AIDS-related symptoms, attend especially to joyful activities of your body, which may be sympathetically feeling stressed as your patients suffer physically.

SUSTAINING HOPE

"Where does your hope lie? Where does your courage to keep going come from?" I often ask people with AIDS in the hospital. Their answers are diverse: "My friends," "My family," "I feel that all this has a purpose even if I can't see it," "Maybe I'm suffering so someone else doesn't have to," "It's just my share of the world's pain," "I know God loves me." Hearing how much hope the sick hold on to helps me hold on to my own hope. Some hope for a cure around the corner. Some hope for one last chance to be at home with loved ones. Some hope in their children. Some hope in heaven. Some hope that because of the vast effects of AIDS the whole world will become a more compassionate place. We caregivers need to ask one another the same question again and again, especially when our own hope flags: Where do you find hope in all this?

In the face of AIDS we find out that it is not just the big, global hope that matters, but the little glimmers of hope along the way: the hopes we have for those who are ill that they might have a more comfortable day today, that a friend might visit, that an intravenous line might last an extra day before clotting, that a person might feel well enough to get up and take a shower or go in a wheelchair to the front door for the first time in weeks. As the small hopes are valued and celebrated when they come to pass, it becomes possible to sustain an attitude of gratefulness that slowly suffuses our own lives. Our patients often teach us that every small blessing of a comfortable moment is a treasure. Gratefulness lies at the heart of every Twelve-Step Program's injunction that we live "One Day at a Time." "An open heart is an infinitely greater blessing than death is a tragedy," wrote Bill, living with AIDS in California.

Hope invested in technology's ability to produce solutions to the AIDS crisis is precarious hope. While patients may appropriately place hope in a new medication or procedure, or their doctors themselves, I find as a hospital caregiver that I have limited confidence in drugs that are so often toxic or ineffective. Hospital staff also tend to see more of the patients who do poorly than those who do well, and we need to remind each other regularly of that skewed perspective. My hope in the health care system lies in its increasing willingness to adopt a humane and holistic approach to healing that appreciates both the appropriate use of technology and intervention and its fitting withdrawal at times, along with an honest acknowledgement of its limitations. Caregivers in company with patients and families need to go through the grieving for fantasies that medicine is omniscient and omnipotent, and acceptance that it is a discipline as much art as science, resting on trial and error, and at best, fallible judgment, and an immense amount of good will and trust. The process is easier for those who believe that healing does not depend on medicine alone, nor is cure or palliation the only kind of healing of importance.

One of the crucial ways we build up each other's hope is by the exchange of stories. The media tend to be quickest to report horror stories: the failure of compassion; the shortcomings of services and science. We read about HIV-positive children being burned out of their homes and turned out of their classrooms, and about adults losing their jobs, and litigating with their physicians. The heartwarming stories of families reconciled, long-term survivors, and individual and corporate generosity and courage are printed less frequently; those, we must tell to each other.

Let me tell you of Frank, embattled with his parents for the past decade because of his homosexuality and expecting utter rejection when he shared his diagnosis of AIDS. Instead his parents cried and hugged him and apologized for the years of anger. "Your friends are welcome in our house," "You are our son and we love you. You can always come home," they said to him for the first time. Let me tell you also of Steve, who brought me a delicately hand-stitched volume of his lover's poetry, written during his final year of debilitation by AIDS as a legacy to other people with AIDS and to his loved ones, bound in beautiful blue paper handmade by a friend. Twenty years ago as an adolescent, Roger had written:

Death is the closing of all doors
Death is the fading of light
Death is peace and tranquility
Death is a flower, closing at night.

Shortly before his death last year, Roger wrote:

Death is the opening of all doors
Death is the walking toward light
Death is peace and tranquility
Death is a flower, opening bright.

There is hope in the sharing of each person's inner healing, even in the face of death.

PACING

Working with people with AIDS may not be a life's vocation for most caregivers; and that is alright. For many, it may be like a 2- to 5-year tour of duty at the battlefront, properly left behind for another arena. Maybe it's most sustainable for those who can grow a garden or raise a child at the same time. The need to change the nature of one's work should not automatically be labeled "burnout." Burnout suggests an abnormal using up of a limited and nonrenewable source of energy. If we feel like rockets falling into the ocean after a mighty thrust (forgive the male imagery!), then we are operating too much as a closed system; nourishment from outside is needed. On the other hand, if we've done a long spell with the desperately ill and dying and find that it is getting hard to do the daily grieving in such magnitude and that we start looking at people on trains and buses wondering if they might have some hidden illness, it may be a natural signal of the need for a change of work. This should be accepted, even celebrated, as a sign of health, not mourned as a failure or weakness. If each of us invests a bit of energy in training others to do our work, then there will be a new and fresh generation to step in when we are ready for the transition.

Even while we are happily at work, keeping a healthy pace is easier if we are part of a helping team. Mental health professionals working from a medical model in private practice may be at highest risk of approaching AIDS work as lone wolves, and may be caught in the rescue fantasy by individuals and families in crisis with their desperation to find help. Needs related to AIDS tend to be so complex and changeable that care networks offer the best hope of helping. How else could requirements for therapy, financial assistance, housing, family support, legal advice, liaison with social service and government offices, and so on, be adequately met?

The task of keeping up with a portion of the literature in the field of AIDS care threatens to overwhelm in itself. I find I can only read so many heart-wrenching articles about gallant young people fighting for life and well-being in a day or a week without needing to lay the whole subject aside for a few days of respite amid my murder mysteries and science fiction.

Similarly, in patient care, one can only be deeply connected with some of the many people in need; others one trusts to the care of colleagues and to God. A colleague in ministry has said (and it rings true to my own practice) that pastoral care of the dying is in some ways like a romance: a deep, intimate connection that touches many parts of one's being and draws upon that sort of energy and preoccupation associated with falling in love. That kind of bond cannot be established with every person or at every time. When a loss comes, either because of death, or because the ill person needs to tighten personal boundaries, excluding the caregiver and others from the close circle, there may be a need to draw in. These are the points that I may leave the hospital for a walk, or hole up at my desk to do paperwork, or even spend my visiting time with patients who require only casual friendly interaction or, being unconscious, silent company in prayer. These are the times I call my friends in nursing or chaplaincy or social service with an invitation for coffee. Guilt-free breaks from care are essential to long-term work of this nature.

At the risk of spending too much time outside the workplace involved in AIDS care, another option both for sustaining hope and for pacing oneself lies in involvement with the community AIDS network. Being with others who understand the peculiar demands of one's work, and collaborating in building volunteer and professional teams for home care and wellness education can offset the intensity of one-to-one care. Organizing and educating are also functional ways of dealing with the need for control in the face of helplessness.

CONCLUSION

It is the nature of AIDS to contain the worst of both predictability and unpredictability. It is still considered a uniformly fatal disease over time. Even though individuals beat the statistical average of life expectancy, they and their caregivers anticipate the eventual outcome. The individual course of the disease and symptomatology varies immensely. Just when I get to thinking I've seen the whole range of types of suffering and death from AIDS (the violent vomiting, diarrhea and wasting, the gasping and gurgling of respiratory failure, the paralysis and dementia of CNS disease, the bleeding and coma, the cancers and Kaposi's lesions), I am presented with something new and more shocking: a young man's infected skin sloughs off from head to toe and he dies of sepsis, laid open to pain and infection like the most vulnerable and disfigured of burn patients. One man dies of Pneumocystis pneumonia on the third day after his first sign of illness, before his diagnosis is even certain; another hovers on the edge of death and miraculously recovers a third, fourth, and fifth time. Caregivers ride the rollercoaster along with their patients, never knowing what to expect next, afraid to get their hopes up too high, but equally uncertain of just when to prepare for the end. There is a special vulnerability that goes with this care, and a flexibility about moving into and away from intimacy as the need changes. There is a special grieving also, not only for the complex histories of loss and anger that accompany patients who are often gay, or addicts, people with a previous medical problem, people from minority communities; but also for the ravages of the virus and its opportunistic neighbors upon the brain. With most other sick populations, relationship between patients and caregivers deepens over time, rewarding both parties. Where the brain is debilitated, relationship may begin to be lost even before death, as the memory fails, cognitive ability diminishes, and capability to receive and process new information and cope with stimuli wanes. The familiar body is whittled away by the changes of disease, and so is the person available to relationship, in many cases.

If we are to sustain our caring for others and our hope for them and for ourselves and our world, we must be intentional about self-care and at peace with our common mortality. Stress management techniques are not enough. We need some philosophical underpinnings for our work, whether explicitly religious or not. We need a community that understands the joys and sorrows of this work. We need balance of vision and activity to replenish the wellsprings of life each day. We require rituals of mourning and opportunities for celebration and for the telling and retelling of the precious stories that are our legacy from others. We need places in our lives in which we are invested in creative and life-affirming and wellness-related projects and relationships. We need to know how to withdraw and rest, and when to stop and pass the work along to others. We need to have a humble and realistic appraisal of the limits of our responsibility. Perhaps most of all, we need to know how to receive love and care for ourselves with open hearts.

There is no way to charge at this work unceasingly and single-mindedly, driven by the sense of bottomless need and insufficient time, without being consumed by it and damaged in body or spirit. With attention to one's pace and balance and finitude, and a gentle and playful acceptance of one's own needs for care and respite, however, it is possible to sustain our caring work over the long term. If we journey together, sharing our strengths, then like the pilgrims of my favorite Psalm, we who go through the desolate valley will find it a place of springs, for the early rains will cover it with pools of water. In the desert of AIDS there will be wellsprings of hope to renew us.

14

AIDS and Spiritual Concerns

Joyce S. Otten

People confronting the specter of AIDS find themselves challenged by spiritual questions. It is not only those who develop the disease, or test (or fear testing) HIV positive who struggle with attacks on their belief systems. So do family members, lovers, friends, professional caregivers, members of support groups, and all who are touched by the problem.

The questions and the intensity of the search vary with individuals. Each person brings to the confrontation the unique background, attitudes, and ideas developed and nurtured over time, as well as cherished problem-solving techniques which have worked in the past. Each person has unique concepts of God, of life's meaning and purpose, of the value of the individual, of the relationship of the individual to the whole, and of a life to come. Confronted by the questions posed by AIDS, most people find these concepts challenged. Sometimes an entire belief-system is threatened or altered.

When concepts change gradually over long periods of time, we may not even notice, but since AIDS often precipitates sudden, dramatic changes in concepts, the wrenching involved can be very painful. After a person's concepts have changed, telling others about the changes in his or her ideas or lifestyle can involve further struggle and pain. "Shall I come out?" becomes a question even for those who care for people with AIDS. Am I comfortable enough with my new concepts to risk the misunderstanding of others? Am I endangering myself, my family, or my friends? What does God expect of me in this situation? Can I meet the challenge?

Because AIDS is a sexually transmitted disease and, at least in the U.S., associated with homosexuality, promiscuity, and intravenous (IV) drug abuse, the death and dying issues confronted by those facing a life-threatening illness are compounded by issues of sin, alienation, judgment and longed-for forgiveness, understanding, and acceptance. Many young people agonize over what and how to tell their parents about their lifestyles or condition. They fear causing their parents pain or incurring their parents' wrath, while longing for family acceptance and help. Parents may seek anonymity, fearing the reaction of other family members or the community, often feeling very alone, estranged, or neglected by God. Spouses and lovers may feel betrayed by God or life, uncertain where to turn, unable to trust. And major differences in points of view may cause rifts between friends and would-be caregivers.

From the earliest inquiry, "Can this really be happening?" or "How did I get involved in this situation?" through various degrees of acceptance, the God questions and the questions of meaning persist for all those touched by the problem—sometimes momentarily resolved, only to resurface in new forms or with new wrinkles. They ask, "What is the point of all this suffering?" "Where is God (or what good is this God I've heard so much about)?" "Am I doing the right thing or the good thing now?" "What, if anything, comes after this life?"

The questions, whatever they are, matter. They provide an opportunity for self-searching and assessing values and beliefs, an invitation to mental and spiritual growth. It isn't the answers of others, valuable as those may be, that are the goal of the search, but the renewal and recreation of the individual. As individuals are reformed and reshaped, all benefit, even when the "how" is not immediately clear.

Although each struggle is different, a brief look at some individual experiences can open our eyes to some of the problems confronted by those touched by the AIDS crisis. Each of these vignettes is drawn from a real life situation. The names have been changed to protect those involved.

A LOOK AT THE STRUGGLE

Jack is a young, bisexual male who confesses openly to a promiscuous past. Now, quite ill, he worries that he will not enter heaven when he dies. Asked what he thinks will keep him out of heaven, he responds, "my sins." Further discussion reveals that he considers adultery the most serious of sins. Since, for him, adultery is any sexual activity outside of a heterosexual marriage, he considers himself guilty. Although he has discussed his situation with his pastor he is, in his words, "still afraid." Jack's many problems are compounded because he appears to be unwelcome in his parents' home. He talks frequently of going home and of his expected or longed-for reconciliation with his parents. But his parents keep postponing the day when they will be "ready" for his arrival. Currently, Jack is being befriended by members of a support group willing to listen to his concerns. He has expressed surprise that these strangers show more concern for him than his family has.

A well-meaning young pastor desires to participate in a support group for those who test HIV positive in order to "minister to the dying." He becomes disturbed when he finds that the group functions in a non-judgmental manner. He believes it his Christian duty to instruct those who engage in homosexual activities about the serious nature of their sin. Because he and other group members do not agree on this and other issues, he leaves the group. But his ideas force those who remain to struggle once more with their ingrained ideas and attitudes. Centuries of social and religious teaching do not change easily—even in the presence of new information and understanding.

Alice began suspecting, even when her son was still a small child, that he was different. She prayed daily for him as he grew, pleading with God to make him normal. But, although her son did not discuss his sexual orientation with her, she knew that her prayer was not answered in the way she had hoped. She struggled alone to accept the reality that her son was homosexual. She confided in no one as she grieved and questioned. Then, when her son reached his mid-twenties, she learned he had AIDS. She berated God for allowing him to be born homosexual, for giving him so much promise as an individual and then permitting him to contract this terrible disease. As she cared for her son through a variety of devastating ailments, she even questioned the existence of God. "What a joke," she thought, "Marx was right. Religion is nothing more than an opiate for the people. It is me alone, me and my strength that make caring for him possible." At times, she saw other sources of strength, such as her husband's help, or her son's courage as he faced his battles. But God? She did not even ask for restored health for her son. What would be the point? A God that does not exist cannot hear prayers. "But," she confesses, "it's awfully lonely when you try to convince yourself there is no God." Sometimes she would think of the phrase, "there's nothing God and I can't do together" and yearn for a God to offer help. The load was too heavy to carry alone. After her son died, she went back to church because, she said, she thought it was expected of her and she felt a need to accompany her mother. But she felt like a hypocrite. Belief eluded her. Questions continued to bombard her. Nearly a year later, she read Philip Yancey's *Disappointment with God*. In his book she found some of her questions and began to think that perhaps some of his conclusions made sense. Perhaps she was not operating under her own strength, but was being empowered by the Holy Spirit. Perhaps

God was present in ways she had not noticed before. Her concept of God and of how God acts began to change. But even as it did, a new problem surfaced. Before he died, her son had embraced the Buddhist faith. If she accepted the teachings of the Christian faith, what would that say about eternity for her and for her son? She is still struggling with her questions, but she is no longer alone with them. She can now talk about them openly with at least one other person without fear of condemnation.

Hanna, on learning that her son was seriously ill in a distant hospital with AIDS-related problems, hurried across half a continent to his bedside. Seeing that her son's hold on life was tenuous at best, she went to a small chapel in the hospital and sat there alone. In that place she "just gave him to God." "I told God to do whatever he wanted and it would be all right with me." This mother tells of many earlier trials in her life and the resulting struggles of faith. Her previous experiences of doubting the existence and goodness of God now made it possible for her to quietly surrender to what she believed to be God's will. Miraculously, her son survives and is healthy more than 2 years after his life-or-death battle.

Pete is Hanna's son. He values his encounter with death. He believes it made major changes in his ideas about death and dying, about life, and about God and the Spirit. Before his illness, "all that" was rather abstract. He wasn't sure about any of it and didn't really want to think about it. Occasionally he would wonder if there truly was a heaven and a hell, but found dwelling on things like that too depressing. His religious background gave him an image of God as loving. At times, when he did things he considered terrible, he would wonder, "What's God thinking about me?" But he never saw God as punitive. Nor was he ever completely convinced that God saw his sexual behavior as wrong, although he was painfully aware that society did. When he suddenly fell ill and learned he had AIDS, he did not talk for 3 days. He simply wanted to die. In the weeks that followed, he suffered two respiratory arrests and a cardiac arrest. At times he hallucinated and imagined that the doctors and nurses were killing him, were witches seeking to cut off his genitals, were calling him "faggot," and conspiring against him. Then he had an out-of-body experience which released him from the pain and exhaustion he had been suffering, an experience which felt like floating around in the presence of a "creamy light." He describes his experience as wonderful, until he heard voices and it started to get dark. He saw something then that looked like an operating room filled with people, some of whom he recognized and others who were strangers. The people were doing something to a body with paddles, and he remembers thinking "This is me! I don't want to die! I have to get back in my body!" He believes he worked at focusing, or centering, himself. Then he recalls a nurse and a doctor leaning over him and the nurse exclaiming, "he's going to live!" Since that time, this young man considers himself a new person. He is convinced that God touched his life when he was supposed to die, that God has much for him to do yet, and that part of the reason God let him live is that God wants him to share his experience with others. "As bad as things can get, God can still turn them around," he now believes and proclaims to others. He is also convinced that "not giving up" and "a positive attitude" help people recover. As a result of his experience, Pete describes himself as more fully alive, a better person, less self-centered, but possessing more self-respect. Although he loves life more, he is no longer afraid to die. A lifetime believer in the power of prayer, he now believes that prayer happens everywhere because "the whole world is the church."

For Jan and Al, the "first death" came when their son informed them he was homosexual. At first, they thought they could change that. When they realized they could not, they were devastated. They grieved deeply. In spite of their son's encouragement to seek help from a support group for parents, they chose to remain isolated. They assumed a support group would try to justify homosexuality. They did not feel ready for that. Nor did they want their friends and acquaintances to know about their son's condition. "We thought people would blame us," they said. Then came the news that their son had AIDS. Now they were forced to deal with all of the issues at once. "The answer to acceptance is knowledge," said Al. He chose to read widely, to seek knowledge through his reading. He needed to "make sense out of it," to "justify it." The books he found helpful were *Parents Matter* by Ann Muller and *Beyond Acceptance* by Griffin, Wirth, and Wirth. Although they originally asked, "What did we do wrong?," Jan and Al now accept their son's homosexuality and his death from AIDS as beyond their control. Although they grieve deeply because they loved deeply, they blame no one—not God, nor themselves, nor their son. Currently, the couple participate in support groups and advise others to do so. They have found that non-judgmental support groups are indeed helpful to those who struggle. "The knowledge that there are others going through what we went through is itself a blessing," they said. And, although they do not always realize it, they are supporting others by their presence. Jan and Al's experience also led them to help other parents by permitting their story to be told in a local newspaper. Fearing negative reaction, they struggled with the request to be interviewed and written about. But they chose to take the chance for the sake of others. They were surprised and gratified to draw positive support from the community—and to find that others who needed help sought them out.

When K was fifteen he lived with his parents in a small, southern town. Knowing he was different from other young men, and frightened by feelings he didn't understand, he sought help by confiding in his pastor. The pastor informed K that, in order to protect others, he would have to tell K's parents and the congregation. That night, K ran away from home, living in subway stations in New York City until he found work and a place to live. For more than 20 years thereafter, K struggled to make sense out of life. Often, the struggle led him to do things he later considered terrible. He always seemed to be looking for love, acceptance and his place in the world. In time, he reestablished communication with his family and delighted in doing special things for his mother. Then came AIDS and a fight for life. He began to attend worship services at a church for the gay community, but even there was badgered by people outside the building who hurled epithets at those who entered. Always he wondered about God's hand in his life. As his health deteriorated, he had several near-death experiences. These he would ponder. What, for instance, did it mean when he was shown the most beautiful stained glass window he had ever seen in his life and knew instantly that that was his soul? What was the importance of conversations with a former lover who "showed him around" in a life that was not yet fully his? And what should he do now? Should he accept the advice of the doctor who told him it was time to let go and die? Or should he struggle to live as he had so far in order to build a few more bridges before he died? The final days of K's life proved a blessing to many as he inspired them to new thoughts, new ideas, and new awarenesses of the complexity and wonder of life and death questions. Concerned that his life would count, he was instrumental in beginning a support group so that others with AIDS and those who loved them would find the going easier. And he found, in those days, friends in the church, including a caring pastor who served him faithfully until he died.

CONCLUSIONS

AIDS brings us face to face with the deeper questions of life. Although the questions vary, and individuals deal with them in different ways, it seems that the invitation to enter the process is universal. If such is the case, it becomes necessary for all those involved to listen more attentively to the questions, whether those questions are our own or are identified by others. If we miss vital opportunities to be instructed by those in pain or confronting death (whether of the body, or of hopes and dreams, or of ideas and concepts), we miss opportunities for personal growth and service to others.

Because "learning" in our culture often means memorizing a set of facts and answers, we may find it difficult to learn to know and understand individuals and their unique experiences (even when the individual is oneself). But help for those involved in spiritual crisis comes not from the facile application of answers, but in the willingness to walk with the one who struggles, listening and caring even when we do not fully understand, remaining present for and accepting of the individual, even if the search seems unduly long and torturous, or paths seem to be constantly repeated.

Those whom AIDS has rendered dependent can also continue to learn and grow by more thoughtful attention to those around them. Who are these people who offer help? What does it cost them? What are their needs and values—and what can be learned from them? If they are fearful, critical, and judgmental, might they also need understanding and forgiveness? If they make foolish comments, might they need better information? If they reflect love and acceptance and compassion, might the love of God be reflected in them? If they bring a new point of view, or a new incentive, to continue the search for meaning and indeed, for God, might it be possible to learn from them?

In the face of AIDS, there also seem to be many questions for organized religion. Does organized religion represent a God of wrath and punishment, alienating and separating by pronouncements and decrees? Or does it represent a God of grace and mercy, seeking every means possible to reunite humanity and embrace the whole universe with compassion? How much of our interpretation of our religious writings is based on a true desire to discover the truth, and how much is based on fear of losing our present concepts? What does justice really mean for a PWA, or for the family, friends, lovers, and caregivers of those who test HIV positive? What can we learn about God, life, and each other, as we relate to each other in this crisis?

Much money and many efforts are being expended in the fight against AIDS. Together we look forward with hope to an end to this threat to life and well-being. But even the worst plague carries hidden blessings. Might the real challenge of AIDS be to discover ways of living together in the world in such a way that we willingly bear one another's burdens, walk with each other through trials, and support each other in the quest for truth and understanding—even when we are very different people? If we were to make that kind of breakthrough, perhaps even those who have died and will die of the disease might count their lives worthwhile.

15

Stigma and Discrimination Associated with AIDS

Mary B. McRae, EdD

For those already considered at risk—homosexuals and intravenous drug users—testing HIV positive can be viewed as an additional social stigma. The issue of discrimination for those who are at risk is often secondary in that these people have already experienced being different from others in a society intolerant of such differences. The purpose of this chapter is to examine the psychological effects of discrimination for those testing HIV positive who are in groups considered at high risk for AIDS. Such discrimination is due to the stigma of being seen as carriers of a highly contagious, deadly disease, in addition to the existing stigmas of homosexuality, intravenous (IV) drug use, and poverty. The factors considered in this chapter are homosexuality, race/ethnicity, and social class as they affect the manner in which a person in the risk groups responds and is responded to in the process of discrimination.

STIGMA

The research on stigma provides a perspective from which to examine the effects of discrimination against those who are stigmatized. Goffman (1963) updated the Greek use of the term "stigma," which referred to bodily marks of disgrace for slaves and criminals. Today the term applies more to the disgrace and the discrediting of an individual or group than to the physical evidence of it. Goffman describes three types of stigma: (1) "abominations of the body," which refers to physical deformities and chronic diseases; (2) "blemishes of individual character," which refers to weak will, unnatural passions, dishonesty, perceptions attributed to homosexuality, addiction, and unemployment; (3) "tribal stigma of race, nation and religion" (p. 4). Although Goffman uses the word tribal, the term in today's society is much more indicative of caste and racism. The issues of superiority and inferiority of racial groups is more salient than their distinctiveness as a group. Thus, white gay men, IV drug users, and the poor have already been stigmatized characterologically; African-American and Hispanic gay men, African-American and Hispanic IV drug users, and the poor of these racial/ethnic groups have been stigmatized characterologically and by race and ethnicity. When these groups test HIV positive, they are confronted with two or three stigmas, which pushes them further toward outcast status.

In Western society, testing HIV positive conveys a stigmatized condition. It has been pointed out by sociologists that chronic illness or disability often become the grounds for a "spoiled" identity (Friedson 1966, Goffman 1963, Zola 1972). While persons who test HIV positive are not classified as disabled and may never become disabled, they are viewed as potential victims, and as carriers who have associated with the more overt disabled person with AIDS. It is important to note that association with AIDS patients can cause one to be treated as if he actually has the disease. It is analogous to being charged equally for the crime, when aiding and harboring the criminal. People who have tested HIV positive or who are suspected of being HIV positive have been discriminated against in employment, housing, and obtaining adequate medical care (New York Commission on Human Rights 1986). Although there is no visible evidence of the disease the targeted person is perceived as contagious and a potential danger to those who live or work in close proximity.

Stigma in this society is very powerful in its effect on attitudes and behavior, and affects both the stigmatized and the non-stigmatized. The stigmatized often accept the negative stereotypes and or perceptions that society holds of them. This situation presents what Goffman (1963) refers to as a moral experience where the stigmatized person has incorporated the identity and beliefs of the society at large and then must use that viewpoint from which to judge himself or herself. While it is generally acknowledged that people with disabilities have their own psychological responses to impairment, other factors such as environment, social acceptance, rejection, ambivalence, and marginality play a role in social interactions (Fine and Asch 1988). Non-stigmatized groups may demonstrate fear and ambivalence in their interactions with those who are stigmatized. Often these fears are based on irrational fears and a lack of information about how the AIDS virus is transmitted. The ambivalence has more to do with the negative stereotypes about the stigma of homosexuality, addiction, poverty, and race. Katz (1981) uses the term ambivalence "to denote a psychological condition in which a person has both positive (i.e.,

friendly, sympathetic, accepting) and negative (i.e., hostile, denigra-
tive, rejecting) dispositions towards some group" (p. 23). The additive
effect of knowing that someone in this already negatively stereotyped
group is HIV positive further complicates the issue and possibly
increases the sense of ambivalence.

Homosexuality is a longstanding stigma in Western society. Until
fairly recently, homosexuality was depicted as a form of psychopathology by the American Psychiatric Association in the *Diagnostic
and Statistical Manual* (DSM III). Political activism on the part of gay
men, lesbians, and their supporters pressured the removal of the term
homosexuality from the manual as a form of mental illness (Herek
1984). While there has been a continuous and persistent struggle to
end negative attitudes, prejudices, and discrimination against people
who are homosexual, national polls indicate that most people in the
United States do not accept homosexuality as a legitimate alternative
lifestyle (Herek 1984). However, the point to be made is that the DSM
III was a step forward in the destigmatization of being gay in this
society. In terms of issues of socioeconomic class, this was a good
example of the power of strongly organized middle- and upper-
income homosexual white men and women. It is also interesting that
groups pushing for the inclusion of racism in the DSM III as a form of
psychopathology have not been so powerful.

Although there is little research on race/ethnicity and homosexuality, there is some concern about the intensity of the stigma of
homosexuality in different racial/ethnic groups and communities. In a
personal interview I was informed that white gay men in New York
City have the support of small ghetto communities and that this
enclave is not available to African-American and Hispanic gay men,
who are isolated from these communities due to race and ethnicity. It
may be that African-American and Hispanic gay men are forced to
conceal their sexual orientation in order to maintain their own ethnic
community support systems (Cochran and Mays 1988). It is purported
that these communities are less tolerant of what is perceived to be
deviant sexual behavior.

In recent years people of African descent have become increasingly connected to being at risk for AIDS. This was most pronounced
in the stereotypical association made between Haitians and AIDS.
There have been several television programs and news articles suggesting that thousands of people in Central Africa are suffering with
AIDS. This type of media coverage took some of the focus off the
white gay male community as being the disease carriers and spot-
lighted people of African heritage as another group of AIDS carriers.
This form of social information provides what Goffman (1963) refers

to as "stigma symbols" which are effective in establishing a discreditable identity (p. 43). Stigma symbols become rubber stamps for anyone who is a part of a given group, so that any man who appears to be gay takes on the discredited identity, even though he has not tested HIV positive and has no symptoms of AIDS. This type of stereotyped association was often made for anyone who was Haitian. Some fear that such associations will soon to be made for immigrants from certain African nations.

The most recently identified at-risk group are the IV drug users. It has been reported that more than 50% of IV drug users in New York City and the Northern New Jersey cities test HIV positive (Watters 1988). According to the New York Commission on Human Rights (1987) 81% of all IV drug users in United States are African-American (51%) or Hispanic (30%). The increase in mortality among IV drug users in New York City is attributed to HIV-related disease; it is believed that this group is subjected to a severe manifestation of HIV infection (NYC Commission of Human Rights 1987).

It is purported by some that stigma is a social and cultural construct that reflects the norms and values set by those in control of the society (Ainlay, Coleman, and Becker 1986; Becker and Arnold 1986; Stafford and Scott 1986). The stigma attached to the IV drug user can be viewed from a social and cultural perspective. The IV drug user is perceived as socially deviant, based on his use of an illegal substance. The manner of drug use, sticking needles into one's body, is also viewed as a form of aberrant behavior. The addictive behavior of the IV drug user goes against the prevailing values and religious beliefs of Western culture. Since the IV drug users are usually perceived as being a part of the lower socioeconomic stratum, they are subject to the stigma and disgrace of being poor and unemployed. In terms of power and social stratification, this group is, for the most part, powerless and has little control over society's perceptions of them. When the stigma of race is added to that of poverty and character, indeed the IV drug user may be more highly stigmatized than other targeted groups in this society.

Some research suggests that the number of AIDS cases is increasing among African-Americans and Hispanics (Friedman et al. 1987). Other research suggests that the increase in these groups is primarily among those who are IV drug users, heterosexual partners of IV drug users, children born from these unions, and the homeless (Day, Houston-Hamilton, Deslondes, and Nelson 1988; Mays and Cochran 1988; Watters 1988). The latter finding could further stimulate class differences within the African-American and Hispanic communities, while at the same time create stronger race/ethnicity and

AIDS associations in the European communities, thus leaving people who are poor, uneducated, and addicted to fight a battle that to some is just another struggle in the vicious circle of poverty. This is a group that is usually poorly organized and has little political power. The communities in which they live are often stricken with high crime rates, problem schools, and poor medical services. If these communities become increasingly associated with having a high-risk group, the community and those in it will become stigmatized as a unit or as a "tribal nation" (Goffman 1963). The issues of power, affluence, social inequality, social stratification, and the institutionalization of stigma become very significant in a discussion of social class, poverty, race, and deviant behavior and require a closer analysis than is possible in this chapter.

DIMENSIONS OF STIGMA

There are several dimensions of stigma that may effect people in at-risk groups in different ways. These dimensions are (1) concealability, (2) course of the stigma, (3) disruptiveness, (4) origin, and (5) peril (Jones et al. 1984).

Concealability

The fact that testing HIV positive does not mean immediate medical crisis and in fact may mean no medical problems for some time, allows the person tested to conceal this information as a way of protecting himself against prejudices, fears, and discrimination. However, concealment can lead to isolation, feelings of guilt and shame, and the constant fear of discovery (Jones et al. 1984). Concealment also forces the person to deal with some of the common reactions to an HIV-positive diagnosis, such as anger at partners (past and present), family, friends, and medical staff; and shock, anxiety, guilt and denial alone (Fernandez, Holmes, Levy, and Ruiz 1989). The dilemma of hiding or not hiding the diagnosis poses a real threat. Divulging this information can lead to loss of job, income, housing, and insurance. On the other hand, concealment denies the stigmatized person the benefits of social support from others who are similarly stigmatized and, at times, postpones adequate medical care.

Discrimination in housing, employment, health care, and insurance are noted in numerous complaints registered at the AIDS Discrimination Unit at the Human Rights Commission. There are several cases reported where persons perceived to have AIDS have not been hired or were refused apartments. In one case an employer transferred and then fired an employee who had tested HIV positive (New York Commission on Human Rights 1986). While the AIDS Discrimination Unit works with the legal and human rights aspects of this problem, there are other organizations that deal with the issues of emotional and social support. The Gay Men Health Crisis and Body Positive provide support groups and information for those who are HIV infected and who have the disease. There is some concern that this type of support works best for middle- and upper-class white gay men. The Minority Task Force on AIDS and other groups dealing with people of color are exploring creative ways of providing support to African-Americans and Hispanics. ADAPT is an organization that deals directly with educating drug users about needle sharing and the transmission of AIDS.

Course of the Stigma

The course of the stigma, referred to by Jones and co-workers (1984) as course of the mark, is another factor that the person tested HIV positive has to deal with. Some of the research in this area suggests that the HIV may remain in a latent stage after entering the body and may or may not lead to AIDS-related complex (ARC) or AIDS (Baum and Nesselhof 1988). There are some indications that stress may be a significant factor that influences the HIV progression (Kiecolt-Glaser and Glaser 1988). The psychological stress of concealment may actually activate the virus while in its latent stage to more serious medical symptoms. A supportive environment and proper medical care at early stages of the virus may prevent its progression.

The other aspect of this dimension of stigma is the perception of the non-stigmatized about the course of the stigma. According to Jones and his co-workers (1984), when the condition is perceived as curable, it is more acceptable and less stigmatizing. The widely known fact is that there is no cure for AIDS. The unfavorable natural history of HIV infection presents several problems to the stigmatized individual as well as to the non-stigmatized persons with whom they interact. Psychiatric literature suggests that HIV-infected patients present evidence of cognitive impairment and affective disorders during the course of their illness (Fernandez et al. 1989). It has been found that the most common chronic mental disorder among the HIV infected is dementia, which causes a progressive decline in cognitive functioning (Piot and Colebunder 1987). HIV-infected individuals often face a number of fears: fear of abandonment, fears about disability, fear of loss of body control, fear of pain and death (Fernandez et al. 1989). These fears and some feelings of guilt affect interpersonal

interactions. The HIV-infected person is often torn between conceal-
ing these feelings for his own protection against abandonment and
rejection, and the desire to share his feelings in order to obtain support and encouragement. The knowledge that one's condition may
worsen increases concerns and may intensify the need to isolate and
put off social reactions of hostility. All of these factors induce emotional turmoil for the HIV-infected person and may lead to affective
disorders such as depression, panic, or psychosis. Thus the emotional
trauma of learning about one's HIV status can negatively affect the
course of the disease process and the course of the stigma.

It is the lack of a cure for a disease that is deadly to 100% of its
victims that poses a threat to others in society and produces another
dimension of stigma called peril (Jones et al. 1984). Peril has to do with
the danger posed by the stigmatized person and the threat of being
contaminated through association with them. This dimension deals
with two primary concerns, physical violence and physical contamination. Much of the research has focused on society's fear of violence
from some stigmatized groups such as the mentally ill (Jones et al.
1984). However, people with AIDS and those perceived to have AIDS
have been the recipients of physical violence as demonstrated by a
number of complaints: gay men have been targets for violence on the
streets; a patient was set on fire in hospital bed; tenants who have
AIDS have been physically attacked with lead pipes and knives to
force them to move from their homes (New York City Commission on
Human Rights 1987). These attacks suggest that fear of contagion can
evoke a violent response on the part of those who perceive themselves
as vulnerable.

Fear of contamination from the HIV-infected can be likened to
early reactions to leprosy and the plague. Although massive education drives have provided information on the transmission of AIDS,
there is still a form of public hysteria when actually confronted with a
person who has the disease or is a carrier. Homophobia and negative
attitudes toward AIDS patients have been found among medical and
mental health care providers as well as within the general public (Faltz
1988, Royse and Birge 1987). Many fear that physical contact or mere
association will in some way cause them serious harm. Several cases
reported to the Commission (1987) indicate this. A woman whose
boyfriend died of AIDS confided in a colleague the cause of her grief.
She was thereafter ostracized in the office and later put on indefinite
leave without pay until she could prove that she did not have AIDS.
An AIDS hotline organization was refused keys after signing a lease
because the landlord feared that people with AIDS might work in
the office space. A gay man was refused medical care in a hospital

because the doctor perceived that he might have AIDS. These are only a few of the many cases reported on AIDS-related discrimination.

Disruptiveness

Another dimension of stigma that is closely related to the course of the mark is that of disruptiveness. It is referred to as "that property of a mark that hinders, strains, and adds to the difficulty of interpersonal relationships" (Jones et al. 1984, p. 46). This problem has been most pronounced in interpersonal interactions with people who are physically disabled. How does one talk to, without staring at, someone who is disfigured or who has had significant weight loss? How does one interact with someone who has made you aware that he is HIV-infected? Faltz (1988) found that counseling staff working with substance abuse clients infected with HIV experienced a sense of hopelessness, feelings of insecurity and inadequacy, and a sense of their own vulnerability and mortality. Siller (1976) refers to this difficulty as "interaction strain." This dimension of stigma highlights the strong aversive attitudes of the non-stigmatized towards those who are stigmatized.

Origin

The last dimension of stigma to be discussed here is that of origin, which refers to responsibility for engendering the stigma. Research has indicated that the stigmatized person is treated more negatively when he or she is perceived as being responsible for the onset of the condition (Jones et al. 1984). Some in the at-risk groups who are HIV-infected are often perceived as being responsible because of their behaviors, i.e., having sex with other men or IV drug use. These behaviors are perceived by some as immoral and the stigmatized person is seen as being punished for his moral transgressions (Gibbons 1986). People who are poor and homeless and HIV-infected are often perceived as lazy and therefore destined to remain in their present situation. This perception of responsibility for one's condition is often a defense mechanism against feelings of guilt by the non-stigmatized (Lerner 1970). When stigmatized groups are not held directly responsible, the condition is perceived as genetic and out of everyone's control. The concept of black "genetic inferiority" has been used as a rationale to account for racial inequalities. Negative perceptions are often attributed to stigmatized groups as a form of justification for society's failure to contribute to the amelioration of their condition.

DIFFERENCES BETWEEN THOSE IN AT-RISK GROUPS

While there are many similarities in the effect of stigma on the various at-risk groups, there are differences between and within groups. Statistically, African-Americans and Hispanics have borne a tremendous share of the AIDS epidemic. While African-Americans comprise 12% of the national population, 24% of those with AIDS in America are of this racial/ethnic group (Commission on Human Rights 1987). The situation for Hispanics is similar in that they comprise 6% of the national population and are 14% of the total group with AIDS (Commission on Human Rights 1987). Much of the epidemic in African-American and Hispanic communities is related to poverty and racism, which has manifested itself partly in the form of increased drug use. The high incidence of IV drug use in poor ethnic communities accounts for the overrepresentation of AIDS-related cases among African-Americans and Hispanics (Mays and Cochran 1987). In New York City, as of June 24, 1987, 30% of all AIDS cases reported were IV drug users (Commission on Human Rights 1987). As a result of IV drug use and the rate of HIV infection in their communities, the transmission of AIDS is occurring at an increased rate among African-American and Hispanic women of childbearing age. These statistics suggest that HIV infection is becoming a serious problem in impoverished African-American and Hispanic communities. These communities are at risk of becoming highly stigmatized in this society. They will fit Goffman's (1963) criteria for all three types of stigma—body, characterological, and race.

Aside from the reported statistical gap of level of infection, there are other differences. The experience of testing HIV positive and of having AIDS is different for people of European descent than for those of African descent. In addition to the issue of race and ethnicity, there is the issue of social class. The AIDS epidemic has caused middle-class whites to incur a number of losses, to which they have responded by fighting back. White middle-class gay men have formed strong advocacy groups to push for legislation and to uphold basic human rights of those who are HIV-infected. They have formed organizations and support groups to educate and to service at-risk groups and their families. This has not been the case for African-American gay men. It has been reported that middle-class African-American gay men lack the support of a visible gay community and there is a dearth of social and professional organizations available to this group (Cochran and Mays 1988). As stated above, African-American and Hispanic gay men may be more private and isolated in terms of their sexuality than white gay men. This may also account for the lack of political and social advocacy for improved treatment and services for African-Americans and Hispanics who are HIV-infected or have AIDS.

For many African-Americans and Hispanics who lack education and who are poor, the AIDS problem is seen as an additional burden to contend with (personal communication, Ronald Johnson, Minority Task Force on AIDS). Many of the IV drug users may fall into this category, since continuous drug use often prevents regular employment. People who are poor typically do not have adequate medical care and therefore may not obtain an early diagnosis, which may account for their statistically shorter life span. The average life span of a white person with AIDS is 18 to 24 months, while the life span of the average person of color with AIDS is 7 months (Commission on Human Rights 1987). People who are poor and who are IV drug users are not organized and, for the most part, lack political and social advocacy groups who work on their behalf.

SUMMARY

While the stigma of race has remained permanently disruptive and non-concealing in this society, homosexuality as a characterological stigma often remains discrete. Being tested HIV positive is also private information that is not identifiable as a body stigma. However, if the variables of homosexuality, racial/ethnic group, IV drug use, and poverty are directly associated with HIV infection, then everyone in these groups can bear a double or triple stigma. A possible danger is that middle-class African-Americans and Hispanics, who already carry the stigma of race, may seek to separate themselves from those in their racial/ethnic group who are poor and IV drug users and thus more highly stigmatized. This separation could be dangerous because it is the middle class who are more able to advocate for political and social change. The overall danger for society is to increase the gap between those of different sexual orientations, different racial and ethnic groups and socioeconomic classes. The fear and stigma associated with being HIV positive can lead to further discrimination against groups who already have a long history of being discredited and displaced in this society.

REFERENCES

Ainlay, S.C., L.M. Coleman, and G. Becker. 1986. Stigma reconsidered. In S.C. Ainlay, G. Becker and L.M. Coleman, eds., *The Dilemma of Difference: A Multidisciplinary View of Stigma*. New York: Plenum Press.
Baum, A. and S.E.A. Nesselhof. 1988. Psychological research and the prevention, etiology, and treatment of AIDS. *Am. Psychologist* 43, 11:900–906.

Becker, G. and R. Arnold. 1986. Stigma as a social and cultural construct. In S.C. Ainlay, G. Becker, and L.M. Coleman, eds., *The Dilemma of Difference: A Multidisciplinary View of Stigma.* New York: Plenum Press.

Cochran, S.D. and V.M. Mays. 1988. Epidemiological and sociocultural factors in the transmission of HIV infection in black gay and bisexual men. In M. Shernoff, ed., *A Sourcebook of Gay/Lesbian Health Care,* 2nd Ed. Washington, DC: National Gay and Lesbian Health Foundation.

Day, N.A., A. Houston-Hamilton, J. Deslondes, and M. Nelson. 1988. Potential for HIV dissemination by a cohort of black intravenous drug users. *J. Psychoactive Drugs* 20, 2:179–183.

Faltz, B.G. 1988. Counseling substance abuse clients infected with human immunodeficiency virus. *J. Psychoactive Drugs* 20, 2:217–221.

Fernandez, F., V.F. Holmes, J.K. Levy, and P. Ruiz. 1989. Consultation-liaison psychiatry and HIV-related disorders. *Hosp. Community Psychiatry* 40, 2: 146–152.

Fine, M. and A. Asch. 1988. Disability beyond stigma: social interaction, discrimination, and activism. *J. Social Issues* 44 1:3–21.

Friedman, S.R., J. Sotheran, A. Abdul-Quader, B.J. Primm, D. Des Jarlais, P.C. Kleinman, C. Mauge, D.S. Goldsmith, W. El-Sadr, and R. Maslansky. 1987. The AIDS epidemic among blacks and Hispanics. *Milbank Q.* 65:455–498.

Friedson, E. 1966. Disability as social deviance. In M.B. Sussman, ed., *Sociology and Rehabilitation.* Washington, DC: American Sociological Association.

Gibbons, F.X. 1986. Stigma and interpersonal relationships. In S.C. Ainlay, G. Becker, and L.M. Coleman, eds., *The Dilemma of Difference.* New York: Plenum Press.

Goffman, I. 1963. *Stigma: Notes on the Management of Spoiled Identity.* New York: Simon & Schuster.

Herek, G.M. 1984. Beyond "homophobia": a social psychological perspective on attitudes toward lesbians and gay men. *J. Homosexuality* 10, 1:1–21.

Jones, E.E., A. Farina, A.H. Hastorf, H. Markus, D.T. Miller, R.A. Scott, and R. French. 1984. *Social Stigma: The Psychology of Marked Relationships.* New York: W.H. Freeman.

Katz, I. 1981. *Stigma: A Social Psychological Analysis.* Hillsdale, NJ: Lawrence Erlbaum Associates.

Kiecolt-Glaser, J.K. and R. Glaser. 1988. Psychological influences on immunity: implications for AIDS. *Am. Psychologist* 43, 11:892–898.

Lerner, M.J. 1970. The desire for justice and reactions to victims. In J. Macauley and L. Berkowitz, eds., *Altruism and Helping Behavior.* New York: Academic Press.

Mays, V.M. and S.D. Cochran. 1987. Acquired immunodeficiency syndrome and black Americans: special psychosocial issues. *Public Health Rep.* 102:224–231.

Mays, V.M. and S.D. Cochran. 1988. Issues in the perception of AIDS risk and risk reduction activities by black and Hispanic/Latina women. *Am. Psychologist* 43, 11:949–957.

New York City Commission on Human Rights. 1986. *Report on Discrimination Against People with AIDS.*

New York City Commission on Human Rights. The AIDS Discrimination Unit. 1987. *Report on Discrimination Against People with AIDS and People Perceived to Have AIDS.*

New York City Commission on Human Rights. The AIDS Discrimination Unit. 1987. *AIDS and People of Color: The Discriminatory Impact.*

Piot, P. and R. Colebunders. 1987. Clinical manifestations and the natural history of HIV infection in adults. *Western J. Med.* 147:709–712.

Royse, D. and B. Birge. 1987. Homophobia and attitudes towards AIDS patients among medical, nursing, and paramedical students. *Psychol. Rep.* 61:867–870.

Siller, J. 1976. Attitudes towards disability. In H. Rusalem and D. Malikin, eds., *Contemporary Vocational Rehabilitation.* New York: New York University Press.

Stafford, M.C. and R.R. Scott. 1986. In S.C. Ainlay, G. Becker, and L.M. Coleman, eds., *The Dilemma of Difference: A Multidisciplinary View of Stigma.* New York: Plenum Press.

Watters, J.K. 1988. Meaning and context: the social facts of intravenous drug use and HIV transmission in the inner city. *J. Psychoactive Drugs* 20, 2:173–177.

Zola, I.K. 1972. Medicine as an institution of social control. *Sociol. Rev.* 20: 487–504.

16

Documenting the Stigma of Having AIDS

David Lester, PhD

There have been many articles in the popular press and on television about the stigma of having AIDS, supported by case studies of particular individuals and by anecdotes (e.g., Ansberry 1987).

It would be easy to conclude that the stigma experienced by AIDS patients is unique to them. We are used to hearing about prejudice against those of different ethnic and religious backgrounds, but surely we are not prejudiced against those who are ill?

Kalish (1966) gave a questionnaire to students in Los Angeles, which contained a social distance scale with questions such as "Would you allow this person to visit the U.S. for a vacation?" and "Would you marry this person?" He found that there was much more discrimination expressed toward all of the physically and mentally ill groups than toward the ethnic groups who are typically thought to experience discrimination. Those who were dying, had attempted suicide, were ex-psychiatric patients, or were in constant pain, were discriminated against more than blacks, French Canadians, or Jews.

This suggests that the stigma experienced by AIDS patients may be, in part, similar to the stigma experienced by any person with a serious illness. To explore this hypothesis, a social distance questionnaire was given to 80 students, aged between 18 and 22, enrolled in undergraduate courses. The eight questions that were asked (see Table 1) were concerned with the social closeness that the respondent would allow with the target person.

Two forms of the questionnaire were prepared. In one form, the target person was someone dying of AIDS, while in the second form the target person was someone dying of cancer. The students received only one form of the questionnaire, unaware that there were in fact two forms.

Table 1.

Prejudice Toward Dying Patients

	Percent Responding No	
	Cancer	*AIDS*
Do you think it all right to permit a person dying of X to visit the U.S. for a 2-week holiday?	8%	34%
Do you think it all right to allow a person dying of X to become an immigrant to the U.S.?	21%	74%
Do you think it all right to allow an immigrant here already but dying of X to become a citizen?	8%	21%
Would you buy a house next to someone dying of X?	11%	38%
Would you be willing to work in the same office with someone dying of X?	11%	50%
Would you be willing to become friends with someone you met and liked if they were dying of X?	18%	31%
Would you date someone dying of X?	49%	100%
If you really loved them, would you marry someone dying of X?	32%	81%

The responses to the questions are shown in Table 1. Two conclusions stand out. First, there is stigma experienced by people dying of cancer. Eight percent of the students would not allow a person dying of cancer to visit the U.S. for a vacation, 11% would not buy a house next to someone dying of cancer, and 49% would not date someone dying of cancer.

The second conclusion is that the stigma experienced by patients dying of AIDS is greater than that experienced by patients dying of cancer. Whereas only 8% of the students would not allow a patient dying of cancer to become a citizen of the USA, 21% would not allow a patient dying of AIDS to become a U.S. citizen. Whereas 21% of the students would not want to work in an office with a patient dying of cancer, 50% would not want to work in an office with a patient dying of AIDS.

Thus, the stigma and prejudice experienced by AIDS patients is real and strong, but it is similar to, although more extreme than, the stigma experienced by any severely ill patient in our society. The extreme reactions of others that are encountered by AIDS patients has drawn our attention to this prejudice and forced us to consider the legal safeguards needed to protect the severely ill. We may thus be moving toward lessening the burden of all severely ill and dying patients in the future.

REFERENCES

Ansberry, C. 1987. AIDS, stirring panic and prejudice, tests the nation's character. *Wall Street Journal* 210, 97:1, 6.

Kalish, R. A. 1966. Social distance and the dying. *Community Mental Health J.* 2:152–155.

17

Parents of Gay Men with AIDS and the Dialectics of Filial Reconstruction

Raphella Sohier, PhD, RN

In the absence of voice and vision, the ability to render differences fades into stark alternatives, a God's eye view or riotous relativism.

C. Gilligan, 1988

This chapter attempts to organize and communicate in nursing terms an emerging theory or pattern of knowing. I have named the formulation "The Dialectics of Filial Reconstruction" (Sohier 1989). It is directed and dedicated to the parents of gay men who are ill with Acquired Immunodeficiency Syndrome (AIDS).

What follows is organized in segments according to Chinn and Jacobs (1987), who characterize *symbolizing* as "the process of identification and the expression of 'what is' "; *understanding* as "the comprehension of the nature and significance of what is"; and *creating* as "the process which involves bringing about new form and/or meaning toward what can or might be" (p. 6).

In order to relate the theory to "what is," one case history (that of the first family with whom I worked) is detailed. The theory emerges as a composite of the interactions of the person with AIDS (PWA), his parents, family members, and the professional nurse. In terms of nursing research, the emerging theory reflects the process and outcome for parents and adult child. There is no intent to disregard the contribution of other actors. Indeed, in the narrative it can be clearly identified that in this case brothers, sisters, and even the children (nieces and nephews) were involved in the process. However, it is the dilemma and outcomes for parents and their gay son that is central to the research, and the cogent factors are those related to meaning, caring, and grief resolution.

SYMBOLIZING

It all began on a Friday evening which I had planned to spend alone, curled up with my cat and a book. Tired from the week's activities, I had just settled down when the phone rang. In a scared and bewildered voice, one of my closest friends told me that his friend Robert had been diagnosed with AIDS. There was a special problem and would I help? It appeared that Robert was recovering from a severe bout of *Pneumocystis carinii* pneumonia (PCP) and that he was insisting on leaving the hospital and returning to his apartment *alone*. On the previous evening he had told his lover of 2 years to pack his bags and leave before he returned. His lover, Jimmy, had been tested and shown to be free of the virus. Both men were shocked, bewildered, and in a state where appropriate decisions were difficult to make and carry out. Robert, who loved Jimmy, wanted him to leave in the hope that thereby he could preserve his life. Jimmy wanted to stay and take care of Robert.

The friend who called was very distressed. He assured me that Robert and Jimmy had a very stable relationship and that he was overwhelmed with the idea that Robert was sending Jimmy away when he was in such need of comfort. My friend said it was clear that Robert would need the support of all his relatives and friends in order to get well and that he considered Robert's behavior bizarre. I remember also that I asked what it was they wanted of me—what kind of help? My friend said that they both needed to sort through their feelings and tell Robert's family about his diagnosis.

Feeling rather insecure about the possible outcomes, I reluctantly agreed to help, not knowing that I was stepping into a new career direction or that I would, in time, become totally committed to the needs of persons with AIDS and their families.

Robert has been dead for almost 2 years. My interaction with Robert, Jimmy and Robert's family and friends lasted more than a year. Meanwhile, other persons with AIDS became known to me and the spectrum of human needs emerging as a result of AIDS has grown and continues growing.

UNDERSTANDING

When Robert was diagnosed with AIDS, his parents did not have certain knowledge of his homosexuality. Working with Robert and the members of the family who did know of his sexual preference, it was possible for me to impact family members one at a time. At each revelation Robert experienced panic. In each succeeding case his brothers, sisters, and brothers and sisters-in-law were able to adjust to the knowledge and respond with love to his needs.

Eventually Robert shared with his parents the news that he was homosexual, *and* dying of AIDS. His parents were shocked, even though they later admitted having "a feeling that Robert was different from his brothers." They also knew that many gay men were affected by the human immunodeficiency virus (HIV). It took Robert's parents a month from the time they received the information about his lifestyle and diagnosis before they could pick up communication with him again. First, telephone communication was established, and gifts were sent with other family members. Later his mother came to visit, and 2 weeks after that, his father arrived for a first visit. Throughout the period I was in regular contact with the family, teaching, explaining, and facilitating care for Robert. It was a time in which the whole family learned about AIDS and its problems.

Robert's parents were simple people from a very small town in Illinois. They were Catholic, parents of three sons and two daughters. They had both finished high school and enjoyed reading but they were fairly unsophisticated and had not before examined the question of homosexuality. The month in which they had known of Robert's homosexuality and illness, but failed to communicate with him, had been used as a time of moratorium. They had read material on homosexuality and AIDS which I had sent with one of their sons. They talked privately and with their other children about the implications for their family and, of course, for their son Robert. It was very evident from the first visit that this child was the Benjamin* of the family. They were all very proud of this youngest son and brother who had achieved so much so early in his life. Robert had graduated from a good university and was working on a Master's in Business Administration. He had an excellent position in a local bank and very promising future, no mean accomplishment for a 23-year-old man.

Robert was not ready to return home and it is doubtful to me whether his parents would have been willing or able to reintegrate him into the family at that time. He remained in his apartment for the next year, helped by friends and community agencies until a second bout of PCP left him exhausted. He had difficulty breathing and could

---

*In the Old Testament story of Jacob and Rachel (Jacob's most beloved wife), Rachel died giving birth to Benjamin. Thereafter Benjamin, the youngest son, was seen as the most favored child. This favored child status makes one "the Benjamin."

no longer provide self-care. He had continued to keep Jimmy at arm's length, though they spoke regularly on the telephone, and Jimmy provided practical assistance in many ways.

Throughout this time I was in regular contact with Robert. At this point I suggested to Robert that he consider returning to his parents' home if they were able to care for him and if they were willing. The matter was discussed, negotiated, and re-negotiated, and close to Christmas Robert called me to say he was planning to leave the city and return to the small township in Illinois where he had been born and had lived until he came to the city to attend college.

CREATING

In the course of the year I had been involved in his care, Robert's parents had changed a great deal. Somewhat aloof, questioning, critical, and sad in the beginning, they had been altered by the effects of the disease process on their handsome son. Slowly they increased their willingness to share in their child's suffering, and as they did so, it seemed that they grew more peaceful, stronger, and more accepting.

To an outsider participating with the family, it appeared that all of the family members—Robert, his parents, brothers, sisters, and brothers- and sisters-in-law—had come to value the special nature of a time in which shared sorrow opened each to the other and bound them together. Because they were closer to my own age and less articulate, I continued to feel some special responsibility toward Robert's parents. I knew that they did not feel free to discuss their family problem with anyone outside of their family and their isolation caused me concern. After a period of negotiation, they agreed to let me make referrals for them to the visiting nurse association and other local agencies so that appropriate support would be available to them in the future. In a matter of weeks, the day was set for Robert's return home.

On the day they came to take Robert home, I went to the apartment with a parting gift and to assist in getting him ready for the trip. His parents had put an air mattress on the back seat of their large automobile. Robert's father settled him gently on the air mattress and put pillows behind and around him, and his mother took a beautiful handmade afghan from the front seat and tucked it lovingly around his body. I asked whether she had made the afghan herself, and she responded, "Oh, no! My mother crocheted it. Isn't it beautiful?" She went on to say, "When my children were small and sick and unable to go to school, they were always wrapped in this afghan." I could only take her hand in mine—I did not trust myself to speak because of the emotion I felt. I interpreted this symbolic act as one which mirrored a reintegration of Robert into the family of his origin, and a willingness to enter as a unit into the time of suffering which lay ahead for all of them.

In the days and weeks that followed, I spent a lot of time considering the transformation process I had witnessed in Robert's family, but especially in his parents. Realizing the serious need for the facilitation of home care for gay men dying of AIDS with inadequate or no resources, and the complications that arise in relation to their homosexuality and the social implications of their lifestyle and AIDS, I decided to study the process.

At Christmas time, Robert's family sent me a card with a family photograph included. Robert was there in the forefront, gaunt and tired, but obviously happy. His nieces and nephews sat on the floor in front of him, his parents stood behind him, holding him up, and brothers, sisters and in-laws were ranged on both sides.

Robert died in mid February, a great bunch of red roses on his bedside table, sent by Jimmy who had gone on loving him until the last. He was 3 days short of his 24th birthday. One of his brothers, both of his sisters, and later, his mother wrote me long letters. They talked about the extraordinary experience they had lived through. They thanked me profusely for facilitating the process that had brought their son and brother home to die. One sister wrote, "Watching him suffer and die, I felt purified; it was at one time the most difficult and the most beautiful experience of my life."

NEW FORM AND MEANING

The poignant experience I had lived through with Robert and his family made me eager to organize this nursing information in ways that would make it available for learning and practice. It seemed to me that this and similar experiences could be studied in order to develop a prototype for nursing intervention with similar families touched by AIDS. I designed a grounded theory project in which I examine the grieving process and the moral decision-making constructs which move parents of gay men to take their sons home for care at the end of their lives. Six parental dyads have been interviewed in a pilot study and the main study with 25 parental dyads is in progress.

The emerging information has three major process steps which occur and recur from the time when parents first admit covert knowledge of their son's homosexuality until the time of his death. They are presently characterized as: (1) antithesis, a time of confrontation, conflict or crisis; (2) thesis, a time of consideration, thought, information-seeking, and discussion; and (3) synthesis, a time of accommodation, moderation, acceptance, resignation, conciliation, and action. Each family tells a different story and the emphasis on the length and nature of separation that follows confrontation, conflict, or crisis varies. In the same manner, periods of thesis or moratorium may be long or short, the deliberation may occur individually, be shared by the parental dyad, or include both parents and the son. Sometimes one parent and the son deliberate, discuss and think through things together, then assist the other parent, or coerce them in changing their perspective. Synthesis may be slow and transitional, varying from a restoration of telephone contact to acceptance which allows common familial interaction patterns to become reestablished and maintained permanently.

As time goes by, the length of time committed to each part of the process appears to decrease and the triad passes through three distinct stages:

Stage 1. Reconciliation—establishment of communication
Stage 2. Reintegration—when the child is invited to return to the family home for care
Stage 3. Reconstitution or conjoining—when the three members of the triad return to a mutually accepting and loving position toward each other

As time passes and the PWA becomes more and more debilitated, the process appears to speed up. The three spend less time in confrontation and thought and move more quickly to considered action. Many families have little time to achieve more than reconciliation supported by loving, considered action. Others, however, perhaps more adaptable in all life's circumstances, demonstrate an extraordinary measure of alteration. The modulating factor appears to consist of the openness and the willingness of the parents to enter into and share personally (not simply vicariously) the suffering of their son. Where parents have the courage to share in the suffering of their child, and as the process steps begin to follow more and more rapidly on each other, the shared experience increases in cognitive meaning. Separation is contemplated with growing equanimity. A subsequent growth in spirituality is inevitable. We speak here of spirituality as described by Fowler (1981) in terms of universalizing faith, not religious commitment.

In a few of the cases I have been privileged to watch as parents struggled with the dying and death of their son, I have seen a transformation, if not a transfiguration, occur. Wrestling bitterly but honestly with feelings of disgust and their original desire to reject their homosexual son because of his sexual nature, they have fought valiantly, and taken him home because the action was mandated by their sense of duty. Before their son's death I have seen these same parents reach the highest levels of psychological and spiritual growth available to them. They have achieved a spiritual re-creation of the original family connectedness. They have progressed to a stage where they could value their adult child as a distinctive member of the human race, a complete adult, valuable in his own right, regardless of his ability to meet their needs in psychological, moral, or spiritual terms. Fowler (1981) has described a similar state, "an augmented capacity for accuracy in taking the perspective of others and in balancing their perspectives with a newly decentrated grasp of one's own outlook" (p. 300). When the triad reaches this rarefied space, they are theoretically classified as parents who have achieved "Filial Reconstruction."

REFERENCES

Carper, B.A. 1978. Fundamental patterns of knowing in nursing. *Adv. Nursing Sci.* 1, 1 (October): 13–22.

Chinn, P.L. and M.K. Jacobs. 1978. *Theory and Nursing: A Systematic Approach*, 2nd Ed. St. Louis: C.V. Mosby.

Fowler, J.W. 1981. *Stages of Faith: The Psychology of Human Development and the Quest for Meaning*. New York: Harper & Row.

Gilligan, C. 1988. Psyche Embedded (unpublished paper), Harvard University.

Sohier, R. 1989. The Dialectics of Filial Reconstruction (work in progress).

18

Help-Seeking Among HIV-Seropositive Gay Men

Beverly A. Hall, RN, PhD, FAAN

Although there have been more than 100,000 deaths from AIDS, this number is just the tip of the iceberg. The CDC estimates that as many as 1.5 million persons may be infected with HIV-1 virus, the majority of whom are asymptomatic (Haywood and Curran 1988). Because high-risk populations are being screened early, many asymptomatic individuals will remain so from 2 to 10 years (Allen and Curran 1988). Most individuals in high-risk groups know from their personal experience with friends that a seropositive diagnosis is likely to result in physical disfigurement and a painful death. It follows then, that having this knowledge, they will have to cope for years with the threat of impending disease and early death.

In comparison to the magnitude of the problem however, there is little research on individuals' responses to living with the daily uncertainty of this potentially terminal diagnosis. The literature suggests that such co-factors as the response of the social network and the ways of coping and help-seeking may influence the length of the asymptomatic stages (Mishel and Braden 1987; Black and Levy 1988). The factors that strengthen an individual's ability to cope with a long latency period and to obtain help and support have not been identified.

As a first step, I conducted interviews of from 2 to 4 hours in length with 11 gay men living in central Texas, who were HIV seropositive, but asymptomatic. Gay men constitute 80% of those infected, and their social networks and support groups have had more than 10 years to form and grow, and their self-help strategies have been shared and honed as more knowledge is gained about coping with AIDS.

BACKGROUND

The model that guided the data collection was Kleinman's view of the health care system as a cultural system (Kleinman 1980). The

166

health care system consists of three overlapping sectors in which help-seeking occurs: popular, folk, and professional. The *popular or lay sector* is the self-care arena, containing individual and family beliefs, roles and relationships. The *folk or alternative care sector* includes providers and treatments outside the professional sector and is frequently classified into the secular and the sacred. The *professional sector* contains services provided by the organized healing professions within the formal health care system.

Help-seeking was defined as any action which is directed at obtaining advice or assistance about a problem or a troublesome event (Gourash 1978; McKinlay 1980; Gottlieb 1976, 1978). Help-seeking is triggered by a variety of factors, including the onset of a problem, interpersonal crisis, perceived interference with social relations and/or roles, and influences from the social network (Roberts 1988; Gortmaker, Eckenrode and Gore 1982). Barriers to help-seeking from the professional sector have been documented and include education, proximity, ethnicity, and socioeconomic status (Kleinman 1980; McKinlay 1980). Additional barriers which may prevent individuals with AIDS from seeking help are the dysynchrony between the culture of the person with AIDS and the dominant medical culture (Cassens 1985), the misperceptions about modes of transmission (Feldman and Johnson 1986), and reactions to the dying (Moynihan and Christ 1987).

The majority of help-seeking research has focused on the professional sector (Gottlieb 1976; 1978). There have been no systematic investigations of help-seeking among HIV seropositive populations. The use of alternative treatments documented in the alternative care literature (Reuben 1986; Morin and Batchelor 1984) and personal accounts of help-seeking (Herron 1984) in the self-care literature suggest a complex area for investigation.

METHOD

To be eligible for the study participants had to be asymptomatic and in stage II of the CDC Classification (CDC 1987), gay, non-IV drug users, and self-reported seropositive (based on a physican stating they were seropositive).

Model characteristics of the sample were well-educated, young, white, and employed in white-collar occupations. Participants ranged in age from 24 to 45 with a mean of 33.6 years. Six men were middle class and five men were working class (Hollingshead 1975). Two men were Mexican-American and nine men were Anglo. Four men had baccalaureate or graduate degrees and five had completed 1 to 3 years of college. Most members of the study group (N=7) lived with a partner. The numbers of months of known seropositivity ranged from 1 to 36 with a mean of 19.3 months. The interviews ranged in length from 2 to 4 hours, were audio-taped, and transcribed verbatim to maintain the integrity of the data and to reduce analytic bias. Manifest and latent content analysis techniques (Field and Morse 1985) were used to identify emic categories and themes related to reactions to testing seropositive. Help-seeking was coded, using Kleinman's model, into the categories of professional, alternative, and self-care. Two raters coded the data independently to provide validity for the coding. A panel of 10 professionals and consumers were then asked to review the coding to determine face validity of the coding categories of professional, alternative, and self-care.

RESULTS

Informants reported a wide range of behavioral and emotional responses to finding out that they were seropositive. These reactions included feeling depressed, fearful, angry at God and the world, engaging in excessive drinking and taking drugs, but most of all believing that their lives were over. The first reaction of all but one of the men was to cry, become depressed and angry, then turn to drugs or drinking. This period lasted from 3 to 6 months. Then they began to alter their attitudes about being seropositive and to obtain help. This change in attitude can be seen in the following statements:

> I had a 3-month period in which I'd get up in the morning, smoke pot, and stare out the window all day. It just came to me all of a sudden that all it takes is just you dealing with the changes. We are all going to die some day. If I get sick, I will deal with it.

> I went through a lot of trauma and turmoil. I look back now and feel like I wasted a lot of time and energy. The most important thing I did was to change my outlook. You are AIDS positive, but you can live with it.

It was not totally clear what factors influenced this change. The data suggested that talking to friends and family, receiving some initial information from the physician, and personal soul-searching all contributed to informants beginning to alter their attitudes. This change of outlook also enabled the study group to engage in help-seeking. The pathway from initial shock to help-seeking was not linear. Individuals were involved in various forms of help-seeking throughout. However, as informants' outlook on being seropositive changed, they engaged in more help-seeking activities.

Table 1.

Professional Medical Services

1. Information about HIV disease
2. Information about treatments
3. Prescriptions of drugs related and not related to HIV disease
4. Monitoring general health
5. Monitoring blood cell counts (CBC)
6. Monitoring T-cell counts
7. Information about health

Professional Mental Health Services

1. Licensed therapist (Ph.D., M.S.W., R.N.)
2. Psychiatrist (M.D.)
3. Minister/Pastor
4. HIV/AIDS support group

A help-seeking scale was developed from these interviews and subsequent panel studies and surveys of 60 men who were HIV seropositive and 10 professionals. Not surprisingly, the most developed help-seeking actions occurred in the self-care sector. A total of 51 mutually exclusive actions were coded as self-care, while only 12 were coded as professional, and 8 as alternative healing.

The professional sector included visits to the primary care physician for medical monitoring and the use of a variety of mental health services. All informants utilized physican services for ongoing monitoring of the immune system via periodic T-cell counts, monitoring of their general health status, and information about HIV disease and general health practices. As one participant stated, "I go to see him and I ask, How am I doing?" Although these men reported having supportive relationships with their primary physicians, they initiated alternative and self-care actions on their own, often without telling their doctors. More than half the participants sought out some kind of mental health services. Seven of the 11 men saw a minister. The use of support groups was low. Some participants explained that some of these groups had very negative foci, and prevented their being positive about the outcome. For example, a 45-year-old construction worker stated:

> A support group that I went to scared the hell out of me. It was a lot of nonpositive types who only wanted to talk about dying. When I left that night all I could think of was, I'm dead.

Table 2.
Alternative Services

Chiropractic
Acupuncture
Massage
Visualization training
Homeopathy
Religious healing
Attitudinal healing
Energy field healing (Reichian, Therapeutic Touch)

Folk/Alternative Sector

Six members of the study group sought care in the alternative care sector. Several of these informants were attending an alternative care clinic, staffed by volunteers, that gave acupuncture, massage, neuro-linguistic programming, visualization training, and nutritional counseling. Some reported that these treatments were used to control the side effects of anti-viral medications, and others claimed the treatments had overall health benefits, including reversing downward T-cell count trajectories. Other treatments, such as therapeutic touch and massage, helped in relaxation and to control stress. Chiropractic, homeopathy, and practitioners who gave herbal medications were used the same way. Many members of the study group were also using audio tapes developed for persons with HIV disease by a popular metaphysical counselor.

Popular/Self-care Sector

Consistent with other studies (Kleinman 1980; Gottlieb 1978; Herron 1985), most help-seeking occurred in the popular or self-care sector. In fact, all participants but one evolved a regimen of self-care.

Self-care actions relied on beliefs about the effects of exercise, diet, stress-reduction, and attitudinal changes on health and the progression of disease. Almost all participants changed their diets somewhat, more on the advice of friends and from their reading than from the advice of doctors. Exercise, especially going to the gym and working out, made participants feel healthy and experience an increased sense of well-being. All of the men reported changes in attitudes and priorities for living, such as living each day to the fullest and keeping a positive attitude toward the future. Some attitude changes seemed

Table 3.
Self-Care

Dietary

Vegetarian diet
Macrobiotic diet
Reduction of meat, fast foods, fat, carbonated beverages
Increase of grains, vegetables

Exercise

Weight work (gym)
Walking
Team sport
Swimming
Jogging/Running
Bicycling

Stress Reduction

Less time in job/work
Change job or modify
Try to get adequate sleep
Keep stress down
Slow down
Meditate

Lifestyle Changes

Decrease alcohol and/or recreational drugs
Take better care of body in general
Change or modify relationships
Decrease partying and time spent in bars
Make self useful to others
Stay busy
Engage in enjoyable productive activities

Attitude Adjustments

Keep positive attitude
Focus on living, not dying
Establish priorities for living
Be optimistic
Live each day to the fullest
Find a reason to want to live
Talk to friends about concerns

to originate from the family of origin, as with 2 men who took their inspiration from the way in which their mothers coped with chronic and severe illness.

Having supportive partners, families, and friends was reported as highly important to health and well-being, but often one or more family members was problematic about accepting the man's homosexuality or the diagnosis. In these cases, stress in the entire family was increased as everyone had to deal with the person who was non-accepting. In other cases, the informants reported that they had to protect their families by not telling them that they were seropositive. Several felt that their parents already had enough to worry about in their own lives without taking on this additional burden. Others just did not want to deal with the stress that would be caused by the parents knowing. Others wanted to avoid stigmatization by not telling, such as the man who was afraid that he would not get to hold his sister's baby if she knew about his diagnosis. In any case, the telling or not telling was part of the self-care routine, because social networks had to be manipulated in order to allow for the greatest happiness and productivity.

CONCLUSIONS

Not unlike other persons diagnosed with chronic and terminal illness, the diagnosis of seropositivity often leads to greater control of one's life and a positive affirmation of the self. Some of the men said that their attitudes were more positive than they had ever been, and that the diagnosis had caused them to have to look inside themselves and find out who they were and what they wanted from life. Many were proud of how nobly they had handled themselves after their diagnosis. Others seemed to have found more peace in their careers and their relationships than ever before. All developed means of resolving their uncertainty and regaining optimism through the development of different patterns of help-seeking, or the development of a new perspective on the meaning of life. Seeing oneself as a survivor, not a dying person, is a key element in this discovery, for a change of outlook preceded taking control of one's life and redefining reality so that re-engagement could occur. Many interventions, services, and friend and family networks supported these help-seeking activities. Almost uniformly, these informants said, "When I die, I will die. I will handle that. Right now, though, I am going to live. I stay away from people who are not into living. I want to concentrate on living."

Thus, help-seeking functioned to obtain information about self-care, and then to translate that information into a positive attitude.

Having a positive attitude toward the future opened up many self-care possibilities that included the range of activities involved in taking better care of one's body, mind, and spirit. What was striking was how successful these changes were in conferring a positive outlook and a coming to grips with what had happened to them. I have followed some of these men for the last year and have in several cases observed how they have handled the downward spirals of their T-cell counts and the beginning symptoms of stage III HIV disease. In all cases, the panic that they felt in the beginning returned to haunt them again, but it was resolved more quickly the second time, and in all cases, it was resolved by relying on the same help-seeking behaviors that they had already learned. Perhaps the long period of learning to live with the probability of early death is helpful in coping with changes along the illness trajectory, and persons who have expanded their self-care activities, have sound relationships with their physicians, and have learned a regime of care that they trust, will do much better in the terminal stage.

REFERENCES

Allen, J.A. and J. Curran. 1988. Prevention of AIDS and HIV infection: Needs and priorities for epidemiologic research. *Am. J. Public Health 78,4*: 381–386.

Black, P.H. and E.M. Levy. 1988. The HIV seropositive state and progression to AIDS: An overview of factors promoting progression. *N. Engl. J. Public Policy 4*: 97–107.

Cassens, B. 1985. Social consequences of the acquired immunodeficiency syndrome. *Ann. Intern. Med. 103*: 768–771.

Centers for Disease Control. 1987. Revision of the CED surveillance case definition for acquired immunodeficiency syndrome. *Mortal. Morbid. Weekly Rep. 36:* 3S–15S.

Feldman, D.A. and Johnson, T.M. eds.. 1986. *The Social Dimensions of AIDS: Method and Theory.* New York: Praeger.

Gortmaker, S.L., Eckenrode, J. and Gore, S. 1982. Stress and the utilization of health services: A time series and cross-sectional analysis. *J. Health Social Behav. 23*: 25–38.

Gottlieb, B.H. 1976. Lay influences on the utilization and provision of health services: A review. *Canad. Psychol. Rev. 17,2*:126–136.

Gottlieb, B.H. 1978. The development and application of a classification scheme of informal help-seeking behaviors. *Canad. J. Behav. Sci. 102*: 105–115.

Gourash, N. 1978. Help-seeking: A review of the literature. *Am. J. Community Psych. 6,5*: 413–423.

Haywood, W. and Curran, J. 1988. The epidemiology of AIDS in the U.S. *Sci. Am. 259,4*: 82–89.

Herron, M. 1985. Living with AIDS. *Whole Earth Rev.* 34–53.

Kleinman, A. 1980. *Patients and Healers in the Context of Culture.* Berkeley: University of California Press.

Lewis, A. 1988. *Nursing Care of the Person with AIDS/ARC*. Rockville, MD: Aspen.

McIntosh, J. 1976. Patient's awareness and desire for information about diagnosed but undisclosed malignant disease. *Lancet 2*: 303–308.

McKinlay, J. 1980. Social network influences on morbid episodes and the career of help-seeking. In L. Eisenberg and A. Kleinman, eds., *The Relevance of Social Science for Medicine* 77–107. Boston: Reidel.

Mishel, M. 1984. Perceived uncertainty in illness. *Res. Nursing Health 7*: 163–171.

Mishel, M. 1988. Uncertainty in illness. *Image J. Nursing Scholarship 20,4*: 225–232.

Mishel, M. and C. Braden. 1987. Uncertainty: A mediator between social support and adjustment. *Western J. Nursing Res. 9,1*: 43–57.

Morin, S.F. and W.F. Batchelor. 1984. Responding to the psychological crisis of AIDS. *Public Health Rep. 99,1*: 4–9.

Reuben, C. 1986. AIDS: The promise of alternative treatments. *East/West* 52–65.

Roberts, S.J. 1988. Social support and help-seeking: Review of the literature. *Adv. Nursing Sci. 10,2*: 1–11.

Spradley, J. 1979. *The Ethnographic Interview*. New York: Holt, Rinehart and Winston.

Wortman, C. 1984. Social support and the cancer patient: Conceptual and methodological issues. *Cancer* 53 (May 15 Suppl.): 2339–2360.

19

Support for HIV-Seropositive Women: A Group of One's Own

Constance Captain, RN, PhD and Florence E. Selder, RN, PhD

Recent AIDS statistics reveal that a growing number of victims are women. Unfortunately, the established services and programs available for women are limited, because women represent a newly identified group of AIDS patients, and the number of women infected has been small in comparison to the two major AIDS populations, gay men and male IV drug users. Surveillance data from the U.S. Centers for Disease Control (CDC), suggest that the number of cases of women with AIDS will continue to increase as the epidemic continues. Concomitantly, the need for services will increase. There is a paucity of both professional literature about AIDS in women and information about services for women. This chapter summarizes the needs of women infected with the AIDS virus and describes the implementation of a support group for seropositive women.

WOMEN'S NEEDS

Women bring a complex set of issues and concerns to the AIDS crisis. Similar to their male counterparts, women face the problems commonly associated with this stigmatized, unpredictable, and often fatal disease. The list of problems is extensive. While the trajectory differs for each person, most experience: a decline in physical and mental functioning, multiple unusual illnesses, the profound grief and loss that accompany a terminal illness, social isolation, fear, anxiety, and loss of basic life supports. The progression of the disease is experienced as an endless, exhausting sequelae of physical, emotional, and social crises.

In addition, there are special problems unique to seropositive women. For example, women who are also mothers must cope with the chronic illness issues such as financial coverage for treatment, as well as child care, their children's health, and concerns of dying before their children become adults. If the children are also infected with the AIDS virus, there are more complicated child care issues, as well as the repercussions brought on by society's response to the disease.

Meeting the needs of any person with AIDS involves an array of complex efforts which require specialized services. In communities where the incidence of seropositive women is high (or women demanded it), programs have emerged which address the unique needs of women. The authors present one such effort; the development of a support group for seropositive women. Their efforts may be instructive to other health professionals and volunteers in their efforts to develop programs for HIV-positive women.

BACKGROUND

With 425 reported AIDS cases (Wisconsin Division of Health 1989), Wisconsin is considered a low AIDS prevalence state. Most persons (58%) with AIDS reside in the southeastern area of the state. In Milwaukee, the largest city in southeastern Wisconsin, an established support group for women did not exist. Seropositive women were referred to the few groups available, which were male groups. Women reported that these groups were primarily oriented to gay issues: informing relatives of homosexual preferences, society's reaction to homosexuality, and advocacy efforts. However sympathetic to the plight of seropositive gay men, these women in crisis found their own issues unaddressed. Frustrated, several women approached the director of a sexually transmitted disease (STD) clinic and requested a support group for women. The clinic director agreed that there was a need for a group that would focus on women's issues.

ORGANIZING THE GROUP

The director of the STD clinic advertised for volunteers who would serve as group facilitators. Interested respondents met and determined that group leadership would be provided by two women with group therapy experience. Group leaders were responsible for facilitating group interaction and guiding members' exploration of their concerns. Also, since a known response to seroconversion is the need for accurate, up-to-date information, two female STD clinical specialists served as information experts for the group.

The group was structured as an open group with weekly 90-minute sessions. The purpose of the group was to provide support and information through shared experiences among women with HIV concerns and management issues.

Given the stigma and social backlash associated with AIDS, it was important in setting up the group to address the related issues of member anonymity and confidentiality. Public service announcements advertising the new service were not used. Notifying potential participants was limited to referrals initiated by professionals from hospitals, STD clinics, and HIV testing sites. The meetings were held at a location without outside identification as to the nature of services offered. Within the group, only first names were used, and the issue of confidentiality was addressed at the beginning of each group session.

CHARACTERISTICS OF THE GROUP

Participants

At this reporting, the group has been in existence for a year. Total membership is eight single women, ranging in age from 19 to 38. Currently, the group is composed of four white women and four black women. Two of the women have children, one of whom has two children in the terminal stages of AIDS. Group members are predominantly from a low socioeconomic group. They are homemakers, blue-collar workers, and college students. Six of the women receive public assistance. None of the women has health insurance. Four women recently moved to the community in order to be closer to their families of origin. All of the women are HIV positive and have not as yet developed AIDS-related symptoms. Knowledge of their seropositive status ranges from 1 month to 1 1/2 years. Transmission of the virus was by IV drug use and heterosexual contact with an infected partner. Four of the women have recently completed inpatient substance abuse rehabilitation programs. This composite suggests a highly vulnerable group of women with very limited resources.

Attendance

In low-prevalence seropositive communities such as Milwaukee, insufficient numbers of HIV-positive women were available to provide a support group model. Lack of a model may have contributed to sporadic attendance, for all of the women in the group attended intermittently throughout the year. Some sessions were attended by as few as one or two women. Since limited psychological services were available, we chose, despite sporadic attendance, to maintain the weekly group format to assure that women leaders would be consistently available on a weekly basis. Furthermore, an established schedule made it convenient for agencies to make referrals.

Deterrents to Attendance

The authors have witnessed a couple of concerns that may significantly affect a participant's attendance at the support group. First, since confidentiality cannot be absolutely guaranteed, a woman's diagnosis may be made known to others prior to her readiness to reveal it. Maria stated, "It took me 3 months to come to this group. I was afraid I might know someone in the group. Coming to this group meant running the risk of my family or friends finding out I was HIV positive and that I also have a drug habit."

Second, seeing others (in later stages) with symptoms of AIDS, is the most common reason women give for not wanting to attend a support group. As Mary stated, "I don't want to see what's ahead."

In addition, several women reported that initially they avoided anything that reminded them of their HIV-positive status. As Mary said, "I wouldn't allow myself to think about it. I'd feel weak and nauseated when I heard the word AIDS." Mary had been diagnosed nearly a year before she sought out the support group. Similarly, Juanita related, "I didn't believe I was HIV positive. I read someplace that HIV testing wasn't accurate. I was retested when I went into drug treatment. Hearing the results was much worse the second time because I couldn't pretend anymore."

Clearly, not acknowledging one's HIV-positive status is a common response as well as a double-edged sword. At first, it is a protective mechanism serving to temporarily buffer a situation which otherwise may be overwhelming. However, not acknowledging an HIV-positive state can be harmful if the woman continues to engage in high-risk behaviors, or if she fails to obtain the appropriate treatment and support. Furthermore, not acknowledging one's positive status may place others at risk if the precautions necessary to prevent transmission of the disease are not taken.

Promotion of Attendance

Attendance was increased as a result of several factors. For instance, when something new about AIDS was reported in the media, more women showed up, as they needed to clarify the meaning of the new information in relation to their circumstances. This was especially true when the information was about recent developments in treatment, such as a new medication. The women wanted to know where to obtain the medication or how they could become part of the experimental studies.

Another triggering factor that brought women to a meeting was learning that their T-cell count had decreased. And, although a woman may have received advice and information during her clinic visit, she usually thought of additional questions after the appointment. At these times, the woman is seeking information and support. The woman may also be in a crisis, and appropriate interventions must be taken to reduce the crisis state.

A final consideration in encouraging HIV support group attendance is the skill level among group leaders. In other words, because there were sometimes sessions in which only one member of the group was in crisis, the leader needed the skills to be able to shift to a therapy model. Counseling skills were needed both to work with the woman in crisis, and to manage the emotional turmoil the crisis might trigger in the other group members. Effective group leadership has a direct impact on a positive resolution for the woman in crisis. It not only benefits her, but also decreases the sense of powerlessness experienced by the other women. Moreover, observing that a crisis can be managed serves to foster future attendance.

Cohesion

Cohesion was a significant feature of the women's group. Cohesiveness is unusual in the early phases of group development, or in groups such as this one with unstable attendance. We suggest that, for these women, confronting a potentially fatal illness generated an urgency about living. The women expressed that life, living, and relationships had taken on new meaning since their diagnosis.

All of the women had similar questions and sought the experiences of others in questions like, Whom do you tell? What do you tell? When do you tell? and How do you cope? By the very nature of these questions, intimacy was fostered among the women. There was a respectfulness in the women's responses to each other. Competition between members, which is a usual dynamic in groups, was never observed in the group sessions. It is posited that this cohesion and lack of competitiveness in the group stemmed from the uncertainty members shared about their health status.

Uncertainty

Uncertainty is the hallmark of living with an HIV+ diagnosis. The sources of uncertainty shared by the group members are: The unpredictable nature and course of the disease, the isolation and stigma experienced, and the doubtful future.

Since it is extremely difficult for a person to confront the uncertain nature of being HIV positive, a major goal of the support group is to help participants manage uncertainty. When women in the group were unable to mobilize and come to the group, other members provided encouragement and support through telephone calls or visits. Compassion evolved through the women's shared understanding of being HIV positive and each woman's anticipating her own future needs. As Joan explained, "I haven't gotten depressed about this HIV thing, but I don't know what's ahead. I'd like to think that someone would come and help me through a bad time if it happens."

The absence of specific information for accurately predicting the course of AIDS contributed to the uncertainty. As the disease manifests itself differently from individual to individual, professionals are unable to define what can be expected of the disease's progression in any given case. This leaves the HIV-positive people without certain knowledge of their potential physical status and what it means. Thus we found group members making comparisons with each other. For example, Tracy was diagnosed HIV positive over a year ago and is currently without symptoms. Marie, who was diagnosed 6 months ago, stated that she feels reassured because Tracy isn't sick. This comparison with other group members functioned to reduce the uncertainty that is inherent in being HIV positive.

INITIAL CONCERNS AND INTERVENTIONS

It is apparent that women who attended the group were at different points in responding to the HIV-positive diagnosis. Their responses and concerns were seemingly based on how long before coming to the group each woman had tested positive. Newly diagnosed women were dealing with the typical short-term reactions, such as disbelief, anger, fear, anxiety, reactive depression, and a need for information, while the women who knew of their seropositive status for 1 or 2 years faced more difficult challenges, that is, the long-term issues involved in living with the diagnosis. Multiple destabilizing pressures were in evidence, such as the effects of stigma on daily living activities, relationship and intimacy needs, existential and spiritual issues, recurrent survival fears and depression, hypervigilant health monitoring, struggles with resolving resentments about the predicament, attempts at mending estranged familial relationships, and in the face of these major issues, maintaining hope and developing health promoting behaviors.

Single women with children experienced unique elements of uncertainty. Concern for self quickly converted to concerns for the children. An immediate concern was the possibility that their children were also infected. The time spent waiting for the results of a child's test was an extremely difficult period which necessitated considerable counseling and support. Professional intervention should be provided to women in this situation. If a child does test positive, the guilt reaction experienced by the mother will require individual therapy. Generally, these situations are beyond the limits of a support group— at least until the shock, anxiety, anger, and initial depression have been worked through.

Women with children who were not infected expressed other concerns. These concerns took precedence over personal issues. The difficult, ongoing task was to assist the women to manage parenting concerns in light of a potentially fatal illness. One of the greatest fears expressed by the women was, "Who will take care of my children if I die?" Her lifestyle in the past often resulted in a woman's being estranged from her family. Her more recent acquaintances and relationships were recognized by the family as transient, unstable, and devoid of commitment—especially to the extent needed. Any expectation that these persons would stand by the woman through a debilitating illness, and take over parenting her children, were correctly recognized as unrealistic. Women in this predicament were therefore acutely aware of their limited resources.

Initial interventions were directed at stabilizing a woman's life and helping her to reestablish familial relationships. The women expressed a need to do this for practical reasons (e.g., child care), but even more importantly because they wanted to resolve previous misunderstandings and realign themselves with their families.

Resources were expanded through referrals for social and health care services. Personal resources were examined. It was important for the women to recognize that their previous lifestyles had resulted in their having developed survival skills. Each woman needed to view herself as a survivor rather than a victim. Accordingly, interventions aimed at reframing situations in more positive ways were frequently employed to offset negative thinking and defeatist attitudes.

Since the women in the group were asymptomatic, their efforts to alter their lifestyles were reinforced. Members reinforced each other's efforts to make lifestyle changes. An urgency about living was often the added motivation for trying new behaviors and taking the risk of using different approaches to resolve problems. The ultimate challenge was anticipated to occur if, and when, their health began to fail.

ONGOING CONCERNS AND INTERVENTIONS

It has been shown that living in the shadow of a potentially terminal illness is best characterized by being in a constant state of uncertainty. This feature of an HIV-positive health status permeated the lives of the women in the group, and served as an organizing principle for ongoing group interventions.

The women in the group attempted to reduce their uncertainty in a variety of ways, for example, by seeking information. Having a resource person who had current information about the disease was very valuable. It was important to correct misinformation, thus allaying many fears that the women had.

Uncertainty was also reduced by each woman's increasing a sense of personal control over her own life and the disease. For example, participating in the group, or choosing who to tell and who not to tell about her HIV status, were behaviors indicative of a woman's taking charge of her life. Since many of the women tended to discount their own efforts, other group members often provided the needed recognition of a woman's positive behaviors.

To assist the women in identifying proactive behaviors, the leaders taught the members to listen to the language each used to describe situations. For instance, Dina kept referring to herself as "my own worst enemy." She was assisted in seeing that this position wasn't supportive of herself, nor was it empowering her to act on her own behalf. Members encouraged Dina to look at how she might take care of herself as if she were her own best friend.

The diagnosis of a socially stigmatized disease that is commonly associated with negative behaviors such as drug use or deviant sexual practices, is known to generate uncertainty about one's sense of self-worth. This was true for the women in the group. Regardless of how a woman had contracted the virus, each woman reported considerable concern about the stigma of the disease. Various depreciatory remarks were used by the women to describe themselves and their situation, such as "contaminated, dirty, lepers," or "I got what I deserved." One woman addressed the group leader, saying "My friends have written me off. Why would you want to spend time with us?" Leaders voiced their commitment to the group by making a point at the beginning of each session to state why they were in the group. This was a way for the women to hear the commitment the leaders had, to them and to the group, regardless of their HIV-positive status. The leaders' repeated practice of making a commitment to the group and to the members fostered cohesiveness among the members. Gradually, the women began to believe the leaders' absolute commitment to the members. Likewise, group members began to regularly attend group sessions. As Karen said, "I believe I matter and I know it's important to be here for others."

A sample of additional concerns expressed by HIV-positive women in the group are identified in the table. As these were discussed in the group, the women received support and information, thereby reducing uncertainty.

Uncertainty was also reduced when the women compared themselves with others in the group. Not being able to locate the initial time of contact means there is no clear way of measuring the disease's status. A woman was therefore able to mark her life expectancy by seeing other women who had been living with HIV longer than she had. In the group, Marcia asked, "How long have you seen someone with HIV before they got AIDS?" Marcia was concerned because she was diagnosed a few weeks earlier and had been doing drugs for 20 years. She said, "I don't know when I first contracted it." Geri, another group member, was in the same situation. However, Geri was diagnosed with HIV a year ago. Marcia now measures herself against Geri and her uncertainty has been reduced. It is recognized that although Marcia's uncertainty is reduced, if Geri becomes symptomatic, Marcia's uncertainty will increase. In summary, the progression of the disease can be marked by a woman's comparison of her condition with the condition of other women who have lived longer with the HIV-positive diagnosis.

RECOMMENDATIONS

One year after the group began, the leaders and members met to evaluate the group and explore possible changes that might improve the group's functioning. The two major concerns that were identified were inconsistent attendance and the group's functioning as a therapy group rather than a support group. As a result, several changes have been planned. The changes are directed at preparing the women for participation in the support group, and creating a more autonomous group. Since these changes are in the process of being implemented, their outcome is unknown.

Preparing Women for Support Group Involvement

Assessment, screening, orientation, and contracting are tasks accomplished through a leader's meeting with a prospective group member prior to actual participation. Women inquiring about the group, or referred by other agencies, are scheduled for an individual session with one of the group leaders. The purpose of the interview is to assess the woman's needs and concerns, and to determine whether a support group is the best approach at this time. The possibility exists that the urgency and magnitude of problems a woman is experiencing may exceed the limits of a support group. These women would be referred for individual counseling or, depending on the circumstances, to other social services or health care facilities.

Several experiences in our group prompted the decision to screen prospective group members. For example, a woman who attended the group meeting shortly after the funeral of her baby (who had died of AIDS) was in an emotional crisis, necessitating that the session focus on her intense need to deal with her grief. On the one hand, it was fortunate that she had the group to turn to; on the other hand, it was a very difficult situation for some of the other group members. Individual counseling would have served this woman better and prevented the other group members from feeling overwhelmed and frightened. Therefore, to protect the best interests of all concerned, assessment and screening should take into account the needs of both the individual and the group.

In the interview, a woman is also oriented to the support group. Information about a typical meeting is given, and issues of confidentiality and anonymity, as well as expectations for group participation are discussed. This allows the woman to decide if she is able to both benefit from the group and provide support to other members.

On several occasions, one woman's immediate needs resulted in much of the group time being devoted to helping her. Interestingly, other group members did not resent focusing on one member's concerns. Either the women were thankful that they did not have the problem, or they felt reassured that help would be extended to them should they be in a similar situation in the future. Interestingly, the recipient of the assistance found the attention problematic. As one member stated, "I feel bad about using all the group's time."

Whether or not this is a problem specific to women's groups is not clear. The literature concerning women suggests that, as a group, women have been socialized to give rather than to receive. Accordingly, women often experience feelings of guilt, shame, and lowered self-esteem when they are the recipients of a lot of attention. Since esteem issues and a tendency to devalue one's self accompany testing positive, the leaders try to avoid creating situations that may further contribute to this problem. Accordingly, addressing reciprocity issues is an important component of the orientation to the support group.

The practice of establishing a short-term contract with prospective members began as a result of the leaders' awareness that individuals, especially when asymptomatic, tended not only to ignore their health status, but also to engage in behavior which was potentially compromising their health and the health of others. For example, several of the women in the group contracted the virus through IV drug use, and had initially joined the group while in a substance abuse rehabilitation program. For these members, attendance at the support group was part of their self-identified recovery commitments. However, once they had completed their program, they also terminated their attendance at the support group. Follow-up contact indicated that these women had become depressed and were using drugs again. As one woman stated, "I can't come to group because I'm using." As leaders, we were puzzled. Had we directly or indirectly communicated an expectation of abstinence, or was this an individual-specific issue?

Individualized contracts with prospective members are now designed to include a statement that specifically addresses their continued attendance at the group, regardless of substance use. This provides women with the needed ongoing support, access to information, and attention to other issues inherent in being HIV positive.

A short-term attendance contract, such as attending four sessions, or calling in to terminate the contract, has several benefits for the individual member and the group. Members who choose not to continue in the group have the opportunity to tell other members their reasons for not wanting to participate. Then the other members don't have to worry about the member's health, or search for personal reasons why a member may not be attending. In fact, regular attendees of the support group do express concern about the welfare of members who have stopped coming to the group. A member may apply another member's circumstances to her own situation, with a negative net effect. A contract is one viable approach to obtaining a woman's commitment to the group and to herself during a vulnerable period, while at the same time providing a mechanism for a member to terminate group participation without causing unnecessary anxiety in or harm to the group.

Structuring the Group for Autonomy

The leaders realized they had inadvertently assumed more responsibility for the group than the members. In examining the leadership, possible contributing behaviors were identified. These are: calling members to remind them of the meeting, starting sessions, stepping in prematurely with interventions, and allowing members to direct their comments to the leaders rather than to the other members.

Table 1.
Concerns Expressed by HIV-Positive Women

"My baby is dying and it's my fault."

"I can't keep babysitters. When I tell them the kids are HIV positive, they quit. I'm going to lose my job if this continues."

"I've moved twice in the past year. Somehow the landlords find out I'm HIV positive and I get a notice to move."

"My family didn't approve of my lifestyle, so I moved away. When I found out I was HIV positive, I came home hoping to make amends with my family for the hardship I'd caused them. I've only brought them more pain."

"It's been a year since my husband died from AIDS. I moved back to Milwaukee thinking my family could help me get over his death. They pretend I was never married and that I'm not infected. I have no one to talk to about these things."

"Many days I get so depressed I just want to get high and forget. It would be so easy to use again."

"I don't know why I bother to stay in school. I probably won't live long enough to graduate anyway."

"The future scares me. What's going to happen when I get sick? Who will take care of my children? Who will take care of me?"

"My tooth is infected. I can't find a dentist who will see me. I don't want to lie about being HIV positive, but if the pain gets much worse I'll have to."

"Telling my family I'm HIV positive means running the risk of them finding out about my drug problem. I can't do that."

Although the women felt that they were benefiting from the group as it was currently operating, they agreed that they did not feel responsible for the success of the group.

A support group, among other benefits, should serve to empower its members. These efforts should reduce negative feelings and restore a sense of personal control to the women in the group.

To re-empower the group, the leaders and members collaboratively restructured it. The members decided to focus on a different agenda each week: information, support, health promotion, and therapy respectively. Members now take the responsibility to telephone other members and to send birthday and friendship cards. Members are responsible for obtaining outside speakers or health promotion films or videos. The women plan to have a celebration night, a time set aside for a fun activity or a group outing. Leader attendance has been reduced to information and therapy nights. A 3-month trial period has been decided on, at which time, the group will reevaluate these efforts. With these efforts, the leaders and members are striving to create and maintain "a group of one's own."

20

Support Groups for the Families and Significant Others of Persons with AIDS

Alan Rice, CSW

Support, as defined in Webster's New World Dictionary, is, "to encourage; help to give approval to; advocate; uphold." Group, as defined in the same source is, "a number of persons or things gathered or classified together." In the practice of helping people in crisis situations, it has proved very useful to combine these concepts, creating the treatment modality known as the "support group."

When the diagnosis of AIDS is made, the person who has been diagnosed goes through a wide range of emotionally-charged feelings, including fear, guilt, shame, anger, and loss of control. The family and significant others of that person will also go through a wide range of feelings, usually similar to those of the person with AIDS (PWA).

This chapter will examine the use of the support group with the families and significant others of PWAs. I have led this type of group for the past 3 years. The information presented here will be based more on experiential information than what the literature has to say. The literature that is referred to, for the most part, has to do with group treatment, not specifically support group treatment. I have come in contact with many families and significant others in my groups and I feel that their experience in the group is the most useful knowledge I can share with the reader.

PROPERTIES OF GROUPS

Groups, regardless of their type, have the same properties. Boyd summarizes four significant characteristics of a group.

The Here and Now Reality

The overriding characteristic of the group, from which all other properties emanate, is its here and now reality. The interactions, the feelings generated, the problems solved . . . are a part of the being and becoming process for its individuals with the present having a tremendous impact on the participants.

Peer Support

Empathic or confrontational interactional responses from peers, those with whom one is sharing a common problem, differ in quality and impact from those that may be derived from the social worker or therapist. The idea that nobody, no matter how empathic, can quite conceive of the experience unless he is living it is supported here. This sense of common experience, coupled with a feeling that others care, can and does impact in the loneliness and isolation that members in a support group express. The group offers the individual the opportunity to become part of a network of social relationships and interactions, and this is a potent force.

Concept of Helper Therapy

Recognition by the individual that he has the capacity to help and give to others diminishes the sense of helplessness and feelings of inadequacy while increasing the capacity to accept help from others in the group. Also, the feeling of strength in numbers comes into play with this concept. In a group, the individual is not alone, which has to give some of the control back to the person.

Group Norms, Attitudes, and Values

Norms may be defined as the explicit and implicit standards for the range of acceptable behaviors allowed to be expressed in the group, stemming from the group leaders and members. This becomes an important concept in a family and significant other group, where it will allow the group members the ability to express wishes and fantasies that might be unacceptable to people outside of their particular situation (Boyd 1977).

WHY THE GROUP FORMAT?

The first question a social worker has to ask is what type of modality would best serve the population being worked with. A group can do several things that other modalities cannot do or cannot do as quickly. A group allows the social worker to treat a large number of people in the fewest hours. A group can act as a screening mechanism for those who might need individual treatment. These people might never seek out individual treatment, but might come into a group situation feeling protected. A group also serves an educational purpose (Berger 1984), not so much from the group leader, as from a sharing of information between the group members.

GOALS

Goals are set in the group by the leader and the group members so that the group will have direction. Goals are usually determined by the type of group it is. For example, in a crisis intervention drop-in support group for cancer patients and their families, the goals are stated as follows: to offer mutual support to lessen the sense of being alone with cancer in a world populated by healthy people, to enhance communication between patient and family, and to inform about community resources (Berger 1984).

PURPOSE

Every group has a purpose for being. Purpose means any ultimate aim, end, or intention; objective or goal usually refers to a specific end that is instrumental to the purpose. In a group the purpose is a dynamic concept, not a static one. The desires and needs brought into the group by members blend together through social interaction and develop into a group purpose (Northen 1969).

The social worker has to be clear about his purpose, especially in a support group. People come to a support group, not for psychotherapy, but for answers about their illnesses which in turn lead to a recognition of their feelings, and relief from feeling guilty for having such feelings (Northen 1969). This is also true for the families and significant others of PWAs.

MEMBERSHIP DETERMINATION AND GROUP COMPOSITION

The particular constellation of persons who interact with each other is an important determinant of whether or not a group will be satisfying to its members and successful in its hoped for outcomes. If a person is placed in an unsuitable group, he may become a serious disturbance to the group, be harmed by the experience, or give up on the support group (Northen 1969).

Although there are many opinions about criteria for group composition, there has been little systematic study of who should be together in groups. Perhaps the most generally accepted principle is what Redl calls "the law of optimum distance": groups should be homogeneous in enough ways to insure their stability and heterogeneous in enough ways to ensure their vitality. This is based on the premise that the major dynamics in a group are mutuality of support and mutuality of stimulation among members (Redl).

Members of groups who share the experience of being in a similar stage of psychosocial development tend to share certain life tasks and common interests. Grouping by sex and age is often useful in providing support for learning various social roles (Redl).

THE SUPPORT GROUP

It is my belief that leading a support group for the families and significant others of PWAs is different from leading other groups. I feel the differences are not that great, but are great enough that the social worker needs to rethink group process.

The first question a social worker has to ask is whether the group is an open or closed group. Is there a predetermined number of people that can come or is it unlimited? Since it's a family and significant other group, is each member of the family counted as one or what their actual number is? Should the group be just for parents of PWAs, just for wives, lovers, and so on, or should it be for anyone that is having a difficult time coping with someone he knows who has AIDS? These were not easy questions to answer, partly due to the complexity of this disease. Nevertheless, I did manage to answer them. The support group that I lead is an open-ended group for anyone that is having trouble coping with someone who has AIDS. The group has no time limit to it, and whether people come or not is up to them. There is no contract made regarding commitment by group members. The group meets 1 day a week for an hour. If I am unable to lead the group due to illness, or if I know I am going to be out the day the group meets, I try to have another social worker there. If not, the group meets without a professional group leader.

Some will argue this is not the best way to lead a support group. Some will point out that allowing anyone into the group hinders group composition. What could a 35-year-old man whose lover has AIDS have in common with a 70-year-old woman whose son has AIDS? They have in common what everyone who might seek out my support group has in common. What they have in common is that someone they know and care for has AIDS. This fact takes care of all the things that would probably make for a bad mix in a group setting.

Group Members

After 3 years of leading this type of support group, I have identified 3 types of group members. The "immediate group member" is a family member or significant other who has just found out that their loved one has been diagnosed with AIDS. This person usually has been in some type of group before and knows the benefits of a group. The "it takes some time group member" finds out about the diagnosis and believes that they will be able to cope without any help from others. This person soon discovers that he cannot cope on his own and will seek out a support group to help him overcome what he believes to be overwhelming feelings. The average time seems to be about 6 months for the person to realize that he cannot cope on his own. These two types of group members make up the core of the group. These are the members that will come almost every week and will benefit the most from a support group. The third type of group member is the "crisis group member". This person will seek out a group in his most desperate time, usually when the PWA has become severely ill or even when the PWA might be in the process of dying.

The interaction of the group with its core members is much different than when a crisis member comes into the group. The crisis member will usually dominate the group because he needs so much at the time he comes into the group. This person will talk for most of the group session and will not be able to give anything back to the group because he is in this crisis period. This person usually will not return for any more group sessions. I once asked the core group members if they minded when a crisis member comes into the group. Not one of them said that they minded or that I, as group leader, should not allow this to happen. Some even went so far as to state that if they (the group) could help someone else in a situation worse than theirs, it made them feel good about themselves. The power of the support group is obvious in what these group members feel.

Stages of HIV Disease and Group Membership

Another reason I believe group process has to be rethought is that you are really dealing with three very different stages of this illness: HIV-infected asymptomatic, AIDS-related complex (ARC) and AIDS. Each stage is different and brings different emotional responses with it. I have discovered it's best to allow the different stages to interact with each other. The person who has just found out someone is HIV-infected is at a different stage than the person whose family or significant other has AIDS and might even be in the final stage. However,

I have discovered that due to the power of the group, these people are somehow able to help each other. It is my job as a group leader to inform the person whose other is HIV-infected that the group might be at a different place than he is. It then becomes that person's choice whether to attend, and continue attending.

Role of the Social Worker in this Support Group

The role that I play as the professional group leader is very simple. I give the group a time and a space to meet. I act as a reference source when called upon, as I am viewed as an expert. I try to allow the group to go where they want to, but adhere to group process by helping them connect themes to help them move on. I very much appreciate the fact that this group is not psychotherapy and should never be thought of as such. I serve as an advocate when necessary.

Common Themes of this Support Group

Many things are talked about in this support group, but there are several common themes that stand out. Control is spoken about quite often. No one knows how much to do or how little to do for the PWA. The group member is afraid of hurting the PWA's feelings by any action that he might take. Mothers of PWAs are afraid of babying their adult sons or daughters and lovers and spouses are afraid of turning into the PWAs' mothers.

Another common theme is the fine line the family member or significant other walks when it comes to hope vs. reality. The group members constantly express a need to be realistic about this disease, the outcome of which is almost always fatal. They also express a deep desire never to give up hope and never to allow the PWA to give up hope either. The power of the support group can really be observed in how the group handles this issue. At one time or another, every group member expresses a wish to give up hope; the PWA is going to die anyway, so what is the point of hoping? The group will rally around this group member, knowing that it could just as easily be themselves feeling this way. The group does allow the person to express what he is feeling, never taking this away. Even the most unpopular feelings are allowed to be expressed, a tribute to the group members and their ability to handle very difficult issues.

A final theme that arises frequently is the group members' need to do things for themselves—and not feel too guilty doing them. Usually it will be the lover or spouse of the PWA that will be feeling this way. This group member seems to need the group's permission to get away from AIDS for a day or even longer. The support that the group member receives allows that member to do what is necessary to be able to continue to deal with this disease. It should be noted here that "AIDS burnout" applies not only to the professional who is working with AIDS patients, but to the PWAs and to their families and significant others. People can only tolerate so much sadness and hopelessness, and everyone needs a rest now and then. This does not make them any less caring about the PWA, it just makes them human.

When Someone Dies

The core group that is meeting has been in existence for about 8 months. I expected that at least one group member would experience a loved one's death. Prior to this group, the core was always small and the group members seemed to have lost their PWAs at about the same time, thus the group changed from a support group to a bereavement group with a time limit on it. One group member's son died and I decided to allow this group member to continue to attend the group, hoping that the group members would support her when she seemed to need support the most. That is exactly what happened and this group member continues to be an important group member while she goes through her bereavement period. My feeling is that she will stop attending the group when her needs are no longer being met. One would think that the group member who is going through bereavement would depress the group and possibly dominate the group because she needs more than others at this time. This has not been the case, as a matter of fact, the group seems to have collectively gained strength from this group member's experience with the death and dying process. The benefit this person receives from the group is the ability to continue to help others, which will help her to adjust better during her bereavement.

ARE SUPPORT GROUPS DIFFERENT?

I believe that a support group, no matter what the reason for the group members' being there, is no different in its purpose. The key to an effective support group is for the group members to feel they are in a non-judgemental arena with others who are in similar situations. The disease can be cancer, drug addiction or AIDS, the premise is the same. An effective support group will allow a person to enter the group in crisis, and through the support and caring of others, leave better able to handle the situation that caused the crisis.

REFERENCES

Berger, J.M. 1984. Crisis Intervention: a drop-in support group for cancer patients and their families. *Social Work Health Care* 10, 2:81–92.
Boyd, R.R. 1977. Developing new norms for parents of fatally ill children to facilitate coping. In *Social Work with the Dying Patient and the Family.* New York: Columbia University Press.
Northen, H. 1969. *Social Work with Groups.* New York: Columbia University Press.

21

Nutritional Support of the AIDS Patient

Cynthia Pike Blocksom, MEd, RD, LD

Nutrition plays an important role in maintaining immune function. Well documented interactions between nutritional disorders and immunodeficiency states have lead to the investigation of nutritional status as it relates to those with Acquired Immune Deficiency Syndrome (AIDS) (Gray 1983; Beisel, Edelman, Nauss, and Suskind 1981; Butterworth 1981). Changes in the immune system have been associated with deficiencies, excesses, and imbalances in iron, zinc, folic acid, copper, magnesium, selenium, vitamins A, E, C, B6 and B12, protein, and calories (Chandra 1986; Dworkin, Rosenthal, Wormser, and Weiss 1986; Cunningham-Rundles 1982).

Research has not yet demonstrated that adequate nutritional status will prevent the acquisition, or delay the progression, of AIDS in those infected with the virus (Bennett 1986), although at least one study suggests that malnutrition may act as a co-factor in disease progression (Quie 1982). Nevertheless, AIDS victims can, through aggressive nutritional intervention, significantly improve symptoms and response to treatment, and help to reduce further immune function impairment.

The nutritional status of AIDS patients is affected by problems of increased nutrient needs, decreased nutrient intake, and malabsorption. Nutrient intake is adversely affected by nausea, vomiting, fatigue, emotional and psychological problems, anorexia, stomatitis, esophageal and oral infections, dysphagia, dyspnea, and pain, as well as by lack of money, skill, suitable cooking facilities, and interest in food preparation. Malabsorption may result from diarrhea, large and small bowel parasitic and viral infections, diminished digestive enzyme secretions, and the decreased absorptive ability of the intestines.

Fortunately, nutritional support of the AIDS patient has recently received attention from a growing number of registered dietitians and other health professionals. Several excellent nutrition resources have

196

been developed for assessment and treatment of the nutritional needs of AIDS patients (Schreiner 1988; Collins 1988; Escott-Stump 1988; O'Neill 1988; Resler 1988). It is also encouraging that many state and local dietetic associations are producing diet manuals which include sections on nutritional care of the AIDS patient (e.g., *The Manual of Clinical Dietetics* of the American Dietetic Association in Chicago and *The Greater Cincinnati Dietetic Association Diet Manual*).

NUTRITIONAL ASSESSMENT

Nutritional assessment, as the first step in nutritional intervention, should include a diet history, biochemical tests, anthropometric measurements, and an examination for clinical symptoms of malnutrition (Schreiner 1988). Patient information should preferably be collected by, or under the guidance of, a trained, registered dietitian. Using the information obtained in the nutrition assessment, the dietitian can plan a nutritional intervention program to meet the AIDS patient's specific needs.

NUTRITIONAL GUIDELINES

Adequate calorie and protein intake are needed to meet the high requirements of the metabolically stressed AIDS patient. Fever affects energy expenditure; an individual's metabolic rate increases over 2% for each degree Fahrenheit above normal body temperature (Schreiner 1988). Energy requirements in the range of 35 to 40 cal/kg of actual body weight are usually recommended. Protein needs are typically in the range of 1.5 to 2.0 g/kg of actual body weight per day, unless there is renal or hepatic impairment. Fluid intake and output records should be kept in order to determine the amount needed for proper hydration. Carrot Top Nutrition Resources has produced easy-to-use, pocket-sized reference cards to assist the health professional in calculating calorie, protein, and fluid requirements (Schreiner 1988).

The use of high-calorie, high-protein, liquid supplements may be necessary to achieve the nutrient levels needed by the AIDS patient. Multivitamin and mineral supplements of at least 100% of the Recommended Dietary Allowances are typically recommended to ensure adequacy.

NUTRITION STRATEGIES RECOMMENDED FOR SYMPTOM MANAGEMENT

Altered sense of taste occurs most commonly to red meat which has been reported as tasteless or having a metallic flavor. A switch from red meat to poultry or fish may be helpful. Choosing other sources of protein such as puddings, custards, eggnogs, commercial liquid supplements, flavored milk and yogurt, cheese and eggs is sometimes successful. Patients may also want to experiment with seasonings, such as mint, cinnamon, and mustard.

Anorexia or loss of appetite is one of the most frequently cited side effects of AIDS treatment. Patients should be encouraged to make a concerted and conscious effort to eat high-calorie, high-protein, nutrient-dense foods as part of small frequent meals and snacks.

Depression may be helped by socialization with others at mealtimes. Pleasant surroundings, attractive table settings, and music may help to make eating more enjoyable. "Comfort" foods, such as ice cream, pizza, milkshakes, and hamburgers should be provided if desired (O'Sullivan 1988). Foods provided should vary in color, texture, shape, size, and serving temperature to make meals more interesting to the patient.

Diarrhea is a problem due to malabsorption and the consequent potential for dehydration. Treatment for diarrhea should include a workup to identify possible causes. Findings may indicate the recommendation of antibiotics and antidiarrheal medications; dietary modifications such as low-lactose, low-fat, or low-fiber diets; increased fluid consumption to compensate for losses; and therapy for lactose intolerance. It may also be necessary to monitor and treat electrolyte and mineral imbalances.

In cases of diarrhea in patients using tubefeedings, suggestions may be made to slow down the flow rate, decrease osmotic load (decreasing strength) and avoid formulas containing lactose. Diarrhea may indicate the use of an isotonic, 1-cal/ml formula instead of a high-calorie formula. Elemental formulas, which are readily absorbed, should be tried for patients with malabsorption. However, this may worsen existing diarrhea especially if formula strength is increased rapidly.

Steatorrhea, an excess of fat in the stools, often accompanies diarrhea. A low-fat diet is often recommended to minimize this condition. Because an undesirably reduced calorie intake is inherent in a low-fat diet, inclusion of medium-chain triglycerides (MCT) oil may be advantageous (Mead Johnson and Co. 1985). Unfortunately, compliance to the use of MCT oil is usually poor due to its costliness and unpalatability.

Dryness of the mouth may be helped by having patients suck on hard, sour candy throughout the day to encourage saliva production. A physician may prescribe artificial saliva to treat this condition.

Fatigue is especially a problem during meal preparation. Fortunately, there are many microwaveable meals on the market which, if carefully selected, can provide a variety of nutritious food that requires little preparation (Greater Cincinnati Nutrition Council 1987). Eating in restaurants and choosing fast foods (Jacobsen and Fritscher 1986) are other alternatives, but these can be expensive, monotonous, and difficult to select a nutritious diet from, owing to limited variety. Having a friend prepare large quantities of food, then packaging and freezing these in meal-size portions can cut down on work needed for preparing a meal by the AIDS patient. Food service programs at congregate meal sites and home delivery of meals such as Meals on Wheels programs should also be explored (Hickson and Knudson 1988).

Getting full too fast can be partially resolved by eating small frequent meals and snacks of nutrient-dense foods that require little chewing. Patients are encouraged to drink most fluids between meals rather than at mealtimes. If possible, all liquids consumed should be nourishing (e.g., milk, juice, and commercial formulas) rather than choices such as diet soda, tea, or coffee. Scheduling drug infusions after rather than before mealtime may improve food intake.

Lactose intolerance occurs when the intestinal enzyme lactase is lacking and is thus unable to break down lactose, the sugar found in milk products. When dairy foods are consumed by one who is lactose intolerant, diarrhea, gas or cramping may occur. Lactase production in the body may be inhibited by intestinal infections and bacterial overgrowth due to long-term antibiotic therapy. Sweet acidophilus milk, soybean formulas, cultured buttermilk, and yogurt are tolerated because lactose produced by the body is not needed for lactose digestion. Pharmaceutically available lactobacillus acidophilus cultures can be added to milk-containing foods to break down the lactose.

Nausea and vomiting may be aggravated by the smell of cooking food. Avoid fried and greasy food by substituting cheese, fruit plates, and sandwiches made with cold meat salads. Eating dry foods such as toast, crackers, or dry cereal in the morning or prior to meals may help to reduce nausea. Patients should consider rescheduling meals if nausea occurs at consistent times each day. Physicians may prescribe anti-nausea medication to be taken prior to meals. Resting after meals in an upright rather than prone position is also recommended.

Pain, soreness of the mouth and esophagus, and difficulty in swallowing are serious problems. A soft or liquid diet that excludes irritating foods such as citrus, tomatoes, and highly seasoned foods may be helpful. Sipping liquids through a straw may help avoid irritation of mouth lesions. A physician may prescribe artificial saliva or a topical anesthetic such as lidocaine taken prior to meals to increase ease of swallowing.

OTHER CONSIDERATIONS

Tube Feedings

Tube feedings are often indicated if oral intake is limited due to swallowing difficulties, anorexia, or other AIDS-related complications which make adequate oral intake unfeasible. Generally a high-calorie, high-protein tube feeding is recommended. Tube feedings can also be used to supplement oral intake.

Tube feedings can be successfully undertaken at home, provided there is education of both the patient and those who will assist in home care. Factors affecting the patient's ability to successfully handle the tube feeding include mental acceptance of the regimen, fatigue, vision problems, and memory loss.

Drug and Nutrient Interactions

The majority of drugs, such as antibiotics, and treatments, such as chemotherapy, that are used for treating AIDS have negative nutritional consequences. These may interfere with nutrient absorption and cause side effects such as loss of appetite, nausea, vomiting, diarrhea, and taste alterations (Schreiner 1988).

Food Faddism and Quackery

Because there is presently no known cure for AIDS, those afflicted often try unproven, fraudulent, costly, and potential dangerous nutritional therapies. Many diet regimens are promulgated as ways to improve or strengthen the immune system. Some of these include megavitamin and mineral therapy, use of egg lecithin, megadoses of amino acids, herbal tea potions, taking injections of food preservatives, restricting yeast-containing and high-carbohydrate foods to relieve *Candida* infections, and following a protein-deficient strict macrobiotic diet. To combat nutritional misinformation it is essential that patients discuss dietary information with a registered dietitian to assess possible benefits or hazards.

Outpatient Care

Many individuals with AIDS function independently for months or years. Often during recovery from an opportunistic illness or during an asymptomatic period, the patient may look and feel healthy. During these periods patients are encouraged to engage in good nutritional practices to assist and help maintain their immune system.

An outpatient nutrition care plan should address nutritional needs, food preferences, supplements prescribed, and meal preparation techniques. Many of the materials used for patient education of cancer patients can be adapted for use in instructing AIDS patients. Support groups, friends, family members, and health care caseworkers should be included in developing strategies for assisting the patient with shopping and meal preparation.

FOOD SUGGESTIONS FOR SNACKS AND MINI-MEALS

A physician or registered dietitian may recommend certain restrictions if the following foods are contraindicated on a specifically prescribed diet (i.e., low-fiber, low-fat, lactose free, etc.):

Cheese on crackers
Cottage cheese and fruit
Yogurt with fruit or wheat germ
Pudding
Tuna, chicken, and egg salad
Cold meat and cheese sandwiches
Fruited gelatin with topping
Oatmeal raisin or peanut butter cookies
Macaroni and cheese
Fruited cheesecake
Buttered popcorn
Ice cream and ice cream sundaes
Trail mix (dried fruits and nuts)
Sherbet
Peanut butter on crackers
Hardboiled and deviled eggs
Granola bars or cereal
Pizza
Fruit salad
Dried fruits
Custards
Peanut butter on raw apple or banana
Tuna noodle casserole
Guacamole or bean dip
Milkshake
Hot chocolate
Fruit pie with topping

REFERENCES

Beisel, W.R., R. Edelman, K. Nauss, and R. Suskind. 1981. Single-nutrient effects on immunologic functions. *J.A.M.A.* 245.
Bennett, J.A. 1986. What we know about AIDS. *Am. J. Nursing* 86.
Butterworth, C.E. 1981. *Some Clinical Manifestations of Nutritional Deficiency in Hospitalized Patients. Nutritional Assessment, Present Status, Future Directions and Prospects.* Columbus, OH: Ross Laboratories.
Chandra, R.K. 1986. Nutrition and immunity-based considerations. *Contemp. Nutrition* 11, 11.
Collins, C. 1988. Nutrition care in AIDS. *Dietetic Currents* 15, 3.
Cunningham-Rundles, S. 1982. Effects of nutritional status on immunological function. *Am. J. Clin. Nutrition* 35.
Dworkin, B.M., W.S. Rosenthal, G.P. Wormser, and L. Weiss. 1986. Selenium deficiency in the acquired immunodeficiency syndrome. *J. Parenteral Enteral Nutrition* 10.
Escott-Stump, S. 1988. *Nutrition and Diagnosis-Related Care.* Philadelphia: Lea & Febiger.

Frozen Assets. 1987. Cincinnati, OH: Greater Cincinnati Nutrition Council.

Gray, R.D. 1983. Similarities between AIDS and PEM. Letter. *Am. J. Public Health* 73.

Greater Cincinnati Dietetic Association Diet Manual. 1989. Cincinnati, OH: Greater Cincinnati Dietetic Association.

Hickson, J. and P. Knudson. 1988. Optimal eating: nutrition guidelines for PWAs. *AIDS Patient Care* (December).

Jacobsen, M.F. and S. Fritscher. 1986. *The Fast-Food Guide.* The Center for Science in the Public Interest. New York: Workman Publishing Company.

Manual of Clinical Dietetics. 1988. Chicago: American Dietetic Association.

MCT Oil, Medium-Chain Triglycerides Fact Sheet. 1985. Evansville, IN: Mead Johnson & Company.

O'Neill, L. 1988. Acquired immune deficiency syndrome and nutrition. *Dietitians in Nutrition Support Newsletter* 10, 3 (August).

O'Sullivan, J. 1988. AIDS overview. *Dietitians in Nutritional Support Newsletter* 10, 1 (February).

Quie, P.G. 1982. *Response of the Normal Host to Infection. Relevance of Nutrition to Sepsis.* Columbus, OH: Ross Laboratories.

Resler, S. 1988. Nutrition care of AIDS patients. *J. Am. Dietetic Assoc.* 88, 7 (July).

Schreiner, J. 1988. *Nutrition Handbook for AIDS.* Aurora, CO: Carrot Top Nutrition Resources.

22

Nontraditional Therapies

Louise Boedeker, PhD, and Anthony Pilla, RN, BSN

We believe that AIDS is not a 100% fatal disease. We base this belief on our own personal experience because we have known people who have continued to live with AIDS for the past nine years. People with AIDS (PWAs) learn to live with the condition by focusing on the here and now and living one day at a time. Their lives are vital and focused on the opportunities life continues to offer. We believe this attitude is essential to health and happiness.

Over the past 6 years we have both worked with many PWAs and HIV-positive people, and we have known people who continue to live, with and without the use of common medical therapies. We are including quotations from PWAs and HIV-positive people to assist the reader in exploring some of the issues involved in making decisions about nontraditional therapies.

Current medical belief is that HIV infection will most likely progress through the continuum to "full-blown AIDS." We have observed that some people continue to live no matter what the medical diagnosis is—HIV positive or AIDS—and that some practices enhance well-being. We will explore these practices in this chapter.

We are not suggesting that nontraditional therapies alone are enough. We do believe that they can be powerful adjuncts to traditional therapies, an active way to participate in one's own treatment, and the vehicle to allow one to follow one's own intuition or inner voice. It is our experience that it is helpful to begin with what internally feels like a good move. Talking with the practitioner of the therapy and being alert to how the therapy process feels are ways of actively participating in one's own treatment. Questions that might be asked are: "Does this therapy seem to reach or communicate with a part of you that is at peace or feels whole? Does your participation in the process interest you? Does the practitioner listen to you?"

We have grouped the nontraditional therapies into three categories: physical, mental, and spiritual. Although these are, in a sense, artificial categories, we are using them as a way of talking about the component parts of a person. Actually, we believe that mind, body, and spirit are parts of a whole, a dynamic unity. We realize that not everyone agrees with us, but we suggest that there is something to be gained from viewing things in this way.

PHYSICAL THERAPEUTICS

Diet and Nutrition

Many people would never put inferior quality fuel in their cars. Yet when it comes to eating, the same people opt for convenience rather than quality of food.

How one eats is as important as what one eats. A clean, quiet, and pleasant atmosphere provides a nourishing environment in which to receive one's food. The food we eat is digested and becomes our body, therefore, the circumstances of our ingestion are important to our health and well-being. Eating slowly, and especially chewing, fully prepares the food for maximum efficient digestion, including more surface area for the digestive process and comfortable peristalsis.

From our experience working with people who are HIV-positive, we have outlined some general principles and suggestions about diet and nutrition.

1. Whole grains are beneficial to most people and can be eaten twice a day.
2. Both raw and steamed vegetables are also beneficial. Over-cooked food and food treated with chemicals lose much of their nutritional value. Raw and cultured dairy products (yogurt, kefir, etc.) are suggested.
3. Minimal meat intake is usually preferable, and red meat should especially be avoided, because of cholesterol considerations.
4. In avoiding meat, however, PWA should be sure to include enough protein-rich foods in their diet. Some nutritionists believe up to 40 grams of protein per day benefits PWAs.
5. Elimination of all beverages containing caffeine is suggested.
6. Elimination of chocolate, sugar, white flour, and preservatives is recommended.
7. Avoidance of iced or very cold food is suggested. The digestion process is eased when foods are served at room temperature.

Stress affects the immune system, and stress-producing foods, a poor diet, overindulgence of alcohol and drugs, all have a price. In addition, alcohol and recreational drugs are now being thought of as co-factors in the progression from testing HIV positive to AIDS/ARC because they can weaken the immune system and thereby increase one's chances of opportunistic infection.

Suggested supplements to the diet are Vitamin C, garlic, zinc, calcium, and B vitamins. Vitamin C strengthens the body's general resistance to viruses and helps with elimination. Garlic is an antiviral. Because of its strong smell people often take the processed form (Kyolic®). Zinc is an integral component of immune system functions. Calcium soothes the nerves. B vitamins aid in healing.

When changing your diet, it's important to keep a food diary. Keep track of what you eat, when you eat it, and the effects you feel that can be attributed to the food.

Edgar Cayce said that "What we think and what we eat make up what we are." Have nourishing thoughts as you eat nourishing food.

SUGGESTED READING

Kushi, Michio. 1977. *The Book of Macrobiotics: The Universal Way of Health and Happiness.* Tokyo: Japan Publications.
Lappé, Frances Moore. 1977. *Diet for a Small Planet.* New York: Ballantine Books.
Reilly, Harold J. and Ruth Hagy Brod. 1975. *The Edgar Cayce Handbook for Health Through Drugless Therapy.* New York: Jove Publications.
Serinus, Jason, ed. 1987. *Psychocommunity and the Healing Process,* 2nd Ed. Berkeley, CA: Celestial Arts.

Acupuncture

Acupuncture can be used as an adjunct to Western medicine. It is the practice of placing needles under the skin at various points in the body in order to redirect the body's energy flow. Acupuncturists believe that illness and pain are caused by the blockage or imbalance of internal energies, and the purpose of treatment is to unblock or rebalance these energies.

> When I first tried acupuncture I couldn't believe I was sitting in a place where they were going to stick needles in me. To my surprise the needles are tapped under the skin without any experience of pain, as compared to the pain in receiving a shot of penicillin.

The thinking that goes along with Chinese medicine is that the person is whole—everything working together, mind, body and spirit. Western medicine thinks of a person in terms of systems, and there is a specialist for each bodily system.

I've developed a relationship with the acupuncturist. She explains to me about health and that the body has the power to heal itself and acupuncture aids the body in that process. Acupuncture adds to my feeling whole and complete as a person. I think that the best way I can take care of myself is by allowing myself to experience the best of both worlds, Western and Eastern medicine. This thinking challenges me to educate myself about my health needs and to make decisions about my own health care: I do this by collecting information, talking with my health care practitioners, praying about it, and following my inner voice, thus causing me to feel responsible for my health situation. This also does not allow me to play the victim while allowing me to experience and express my own power over myself.

SUGGESTED READING

Kaptchuk, Ted J. 1983. *The Web That Has No Weaver*. New York: Congdon & Weed.
Manaka, Yoshio, et al. 1972. *The Layman's Guide to Acupuncture*. New York and Tokyo: Weatherhill.
Mitchel, Ellinor. 1987. *Plain Talk About Acupuncture*. New York: Whalehall Publishers.
Rabinowitz, Naomi. 1987. Acupuncture and the AIDS epidemic: reflections on the treatment of 200 patients in four years. *Am. J. Acupuncture* 15, 1 (January-March).
Smith, Michael O. 1988. AIDS: Results of Chinese medical treatment show frequent symptom relief and some apparent long-term remissions. *Am. J. Acupuncture* 16, 2, (April-June).

Body Work

"I feel at home again" is one comment that is made after some form of body work. It could be reiki, shiatsu massage, or Swedish massage (descriptions of each are found at the end of this section). What often happens is that people with health issues spend more time living "in their heads" than living in their entire bodies. Sometimes it appears that the body is the enemy or the "problem," and must be watched for symptoms.

Another related issue is that some people with AIDS or ARC become less physical with others. Touching and being touched often serve as powerful stress reducers and pleasure creators. Being cared for by someone else and touched in a supportive way often increases a sense of well-being. Sometimes people with lesions begin to feel disgusted by their bodies. To experience someone touching them in a loving way may encourage self acceptance.

The quieting of the mind that happens during body work is often that much-needed rest from thinking, "What should I be doing? Am I doing enough? What if?" etc.

Learning to do body work techniques on oneself is empowering. It also gives one something to pass on to another and is a way of making connections with others.

Reiki is an Oriental term that means "universal life force energy." By holding his or her hands close to but not touching the receiver's body, the reiki practitioner is said to activate and balance the life force energy. The techniques focus on the contacting of the energy field or aura around the body. This therapy is used for mental distress, chronic and acute physical problems, and is thought to enhance the function of the lymph system.

Shiatsu is a Japanese word meaning finger pressure. It is also called acupressure and is sometimes thought of as acupuncture without needles. Varying degrees of finger pressure are used to balance the life energy that flows through the body. After a shiatsu session people often report achieving a meditative, peaceful state. One optimal benefit is that shiatsu, like acupuncture, strengthens the lymph system.

Swedish massage consists of manipulations and long strokes that soothe the peripheral nerves and skeletal muscles and enhance general circulation. It, too, is thought to enhance the lymph function. Swedish massage assists the body's healing process by stimulating the elimination of toxins and facilitating the nutrition of tissues as well as producing an overall state of deep relaxation.

We talk about these forms of body work as if they are separate and discrete. Actually, the same general effect may be produced by all.

SUGGESTED READING

Maanum, Armand and Herb Montgomery. 1985. *Complete Book of Swedish Massage*. New York: Harper & Row.
Ohashi, Wataru. 1976. *Do It Yourself Shiatsu*. Vicki Lindner, ed. New York: E.P. Dutton.
Ray, Barbara. 1983. *The Reiki Factor*. St. Petersburg, FL: Radiance Associates.
Masunaga, Shizuto with Wataru Ohashi. 1977. *Zen Shiatsu*. Tokyo: Japan Publications.

Exercise

Most of us know the joy and feeling of well-being that comes from exercise. We eat with more enthusiasm, sleep with more ease, and move with more elasticity and vigor. There are many forms of exercise and body movement. We have chosen to focus on the practice of Hatha Yoga. Hatha Yoga has been used for years in Asia as a way to develop and maintain a flexible body and to strengthen immunity. In contrast to gymnastic exercises, Hatha Yoga emphasizes smoothness of movement and ease of muscle stretching. It is helpful for releasing tensions, balancing the energy throughout the body, and increasing the flexibility of the spine.

The slow, connected movements of yoga emphasize the body as a total system. Doing this form of exercise properly enables one to feel connected, refreshed, and tranquil. Hatha Yoga is a way of physical training to prepare the mind and body for meditation.

SUGGESTED READING

Gach, Michael Reed, with Carolyn Marco. 1981. *Acu-Yoga: The Acupressure Stress Management Book.* Tokyo: Japan Publications.
Carr, Rachel. 1972. *Yoga for All Ages.* New York: Fireside Publications.
Masahiro Oki. 1977. *Healing Yourself Through Okido Yoga.* Tokyo: Japan Publications.

MENTAL THERAPEUTICS

Talk Therapy

The scope of talk therapy is broad and includes individual counseling, psychotherapy, primal therapy, group therapy, as well as support groups, Twelve-Step programs, and so forth. We have consolidated aspects of many forms of talk therapy in order to show the benefits of speaking about one's own thoughts and feelings. One person's experience with talk therapy will illustrate this.

In 1984, I went for a check-up because at that time there was a lot of talk about AIDS. Previously, I had been an IV drug user and into anonymous sex with numerous men, which meant that I was in a high-risk group for the virus. At that time I was diagnosed with thrush, a yeast infection of the mouth commonly found in people with the virus. From that time until I was diagnosed with AIDS in 1986, I lived with fear and anxiety about AIDS and I didn't talk much about it in hopes that it would just go away.

When I was diagnosed with AIDS I was relieved to find out that I wouldn't die immediately. Then I realized I had a choice: either I could learn how to live with AIDS or I could wait and die. I chose to live with the condition of AIDS. After choosing to live I found that I needed to educate myself about the virus and how it operates. I also read books such as *Love, Medicine and Miracles,* by Bernie Siegel; *The Anatomy of an Illness,* by Norman Cousins; and *You Can Heal Your Life,* by Louise Hay. These books opened my mind to how I might live with AIDS. I also began talking with others who had the same condition to learn how they were dealing with the virus. By talking with others I developed the attitude, if others can live and be happy with a life-threatening illness, so can I.

I spent most of my life emotionally isolated from people. After I found out that I had AIDS, I went to my therapy group and started talking about how I was feeling and this began the end of my emotional isolation. Now I started to feel more alive than when I didn't have AIDS! Feelings of anger, rage, sorrow, fear, and anxiety were common when I was first aware of having the virus. Talking about these feelings, whether it be with a close friend, a therapist, in a group therapy situation, a support group or a Twelve-Step meeting, allowed me to feel better about myself. I also believe that holding onto these emotions and not expressing them can cause harm to the immune system, and expressing them and letting go of them can enhance it. Today I am very interested in reading about and experiencing the effect that emotions and attitudes play in relation to our immune system.

As I mentioned before, anger was my first reaction to the diagnosis of having the virus. I began to learn how to express my anger in a constructive way. For me, this meant allowing myself to let the other members in the therapy group know how angry I was. This was probably one of the scariest things I've done. But I am here to say that I got through the experience and am a better person for it!

Because I am in recovery from addiction, I attend Twelve-Step meetings for recovering addicts who are HIV positive AIDS/ARC. Here we all talk about how we are handling the diagnosis. One thing that I have observed is that people who are in Twelve-Step programs tend to be more accepting of their situations. I've noticed that when a member of the group becomes ill, he or she is surrounded by people while in the hospital. Opening up and talking to people about our experience allows us to be there for people and for others to be there for us.

When I was in the hospital with my first episode of PCP (*Pneumocystis carinii* pneumonia) I had people in to visit every day. One of the things that touched me about this was that I wasn't alone and that I could really count on others to be there. This was not always the case in my life. I came from a place of addiction, backroom bars, and bath houses. The only time that people communicated was to solicit drugs or sex. AIDS has given me the opportunity to begin to know who I am, my thoughts and feelings, and to begin to identify and explore these with others by using talk therapy.

SPIRITUAL THERAPEUTICS

Concepts of God, religion, and spirituality are for many of us unpleasant, repressive associations from childhood. Such a perspective notwithstanding, there are other ideas about spirituality that can be tremendously supportive and even transforming. There are countless perspectives on spirit and spirituality, ranging from various organized religious practices to individual observances, and employ such techniques as meditation, prayer, chanting, and the use of crystals and affirmations. Two ideas, metaphysics and higher power, are developed here.

Metaphysics

Metaphysicians believe that our thought is creative and powerful—what we think we attract to us. If our tendency is to think we are separate and alone, we will create those situations in our lives. It also follows that what we think we can unthink. If we have created unpleasant conditions as a result of our thinking, we can reverse our situations by changing how and what we think.

Willis Kinnear's book *30-Day Mental Diet* recommends we pay attention to the kinds of thoughts we allow in and retain. He asserts that our thoughts often determine the functioning and the health of our physical bodies, as well as the state of our relationships with others, and the degree of success which we may be able to achieve.

SUGGESTED READING

Hay, Louise L. 1984. *You Can Heal Your Life*. Santa Monica, CA: Hay House.
Holmes, Ernest. 1938. *The Science of Mind*. New York: Dodd, Mead.
Kinnear, Willis. 1984. *30-Day Mental Diet*. Los Angeles: Science of Mind Publications.
The AIDS Book. 1988. Santa Monica, CA: Hay House.

Higher Power

Believers in a higher power accept that a central force exists in the universe which guides them through life. This force has been given many names. The point is that belief in a higher power enables believers to act and feel in ways beyond what had earlier seemed possible to them. By merging with the universe and surrendering to a power greater than oneself the individual acknowledges that he can't control everything and that the results are in the hands of a higher power. For example, we may be frozen with fear and our conscious contact with a power greater than ourselves can help us move through our fear and thereby transform the fear into faith. Here is a story of how belief in a higher power works in the life of one PWA.

> I was raised Catholic and I believed that God was something outside of me. I was taught that I would be acceptable to God if I did certain things. Well, I never felt that I measured up to what the Church taught me. When I started to have feelings of homosexuality, I prayed that God would remove them. Well, they weren't removed; I got angry at God and set the idea of God on the shelf. I was ashamed and guilty for having these homosexual feelings. Also, the message I received from society about homosexuality was negative, allowing me to feel I wasn't worthy of love from a higher power.
> A short while after I was diagnosed with AIDS I spoke to a person who had been asymptomatic for a couple of years. When I asked him

to what he thought he owed his state of health, he told me that he did what his doctors told him to do, he ate well and exercised daily, and whatever was too much to handle he turned over to his higher power. He said he learned to contact that place inside of himself that was in touch with a power greater than himself alone. I knew what he was talking about; to me this means to follow my inner voice.

Coming to believe in a higher power helps me through the rough times. Recently, I have experienced severe headaches. This has been going on for about 9 months. Because I have had AIDS for the past 2 years, having the headaches caused me a lot of anxiety and fear. You see, even though I have AIDS I still live a full and productive life. I have been sick twice. Once with PCP and the second time with a bacterial infection. Since my second bout of illness I have been free of infection and other symptoms.

When I started to experience headaches I had tests done, including a spinal tap, and a CAT scan of the brain. Both were negative. I also went to an ear, nose and throat specialist, and had sinus x-rays. Then I was treated for sinus infections with antibiotics. As the headaches still persisted, I then tried acupuncture and I received some relief from the pain, although the problem still persisted in cycles. I then stopped all medications based on the idea that I could be having a reaction to AZT or Acyclovir, the two medications I take for my condition. I even went to an allergist and was tested for allergies. The allergist said I was allergic to dust, but that he would not treat me with immunotherapy because he didn't feel safe about stimulating my immune system. I have finally traced the cause of the headaches by noting that they occur every 2 weeks, persisting for about 5 to 7 days, and then clear up. This coincides with the use of Pentamadine, an aerosal mist used to prevent PCP.

Belief in a higher power has helped me to continue looking for the cause of my physical pain. I didn't give up but I did surrender my attempt at controlling the situation. I asked my higher power to give me the courage to take the next step. During this time I continued to work at my job, socialize with my friends, play with my animals and complete course work at school. I know that if I didn't have a belief in a higher power I would have felt the headaches were too much to go through and I would have hoped to die.

I went to a Christian Science practitioner and she told me that God's love is like the sun—it shines everywhere and I am the one who walks through life with an umbrella, shadowing God's love from me. I have a choice to stay in the shadow or receive the love.

Since my diagnosis of AIDS I have to deal with my feelings and thoughts about death and dying. I am afraid of the dying process more so than death itself. I have read books about death and dying so I might begin to gain a perspective on death. My understanding of death today is that it is not a matter of winning or losing, it just is.

SUGGESTED READING

Eddy, Mary Baker. 1971. *Science and Health with a Key to the Scriptures*. Boston: First Church of Christ, Scientist.
Foulks, Frances W. 1985. *Effectual Prayer*. Unity Village, MO: Unity Books.

Foundation for Inner Peace. 1975. *A Course in Miracles.* Farmingdale, NY: Coleman Graphics.

Holmes, Ernest. 1985. *How to Change Your Life.* Los Angeles: Dodd, Mead.

McCall, Fr. Peter and Maryanne Lacey. 1985. *An Invitation to Healing.* Yonkers, NY: Peace of Christ Prayer Ministry.

Roth, Charles. *More Power to You.* 1982. Unity Village, MO: Unity Books.

NEXT STEPS

Life is not a technique and the process of living is more than adding together some mind plus some body plus some spirit. Mind, body, and spirit cooperate. Just as the fingers and thumb together accomplish something more and something different from the actions of each member, so too do body, mind, and spirit. The connection of the body to the earth, the connection of the mind to larger thoughts, and the connection of the spirit to all that is, creates a universe within a universe. Krishnamurti wrote *You Are the World* in which he says, "In oneself lies the whole world, and if you know how to look and learn, then the door is there and the key is in your hand. Nobody on earth can give you either that key or the door to open, except yourself." Does this sound interesting to you?

We believe that techniques can help you learn about yourself and help you connect with others. We suggest that you work with others who support you. If that means organized religion, that's fine. If it means exploring new areas to you such as Christian Science or Science of Mind, then try that. There are support groups such as the Healing Circle in New York City and the Louise Hay groups in California. Throughout the U.S. and Canada there are Twelve-Step groups for people in recovery from co-dependent relationships, drug addiction, alcohol addiction, compulsive sex addiction, food addiction, addiction to gambling, and emotional addiction.

If you are in an isolated area or an area where there is a lot of fear and misunderstanding about HIV infection and AIDS, you can start by doing reading that sounds promising. We also encourage you to write to Dr. Louise Boedeker in care of the publisher of this book.

People have experienced two roads with AIDS and HIV infection, acceptance or despair. Most people see it as a death sentence. If you follow that line of thinking, then simply being born can also be seen as a death sentence. AIDS and HIV infection can also be seen as an opportunity for growth. In this context, health and happiness are not produced by situations but they are produced by one's own mind. Through the process of meditation and visualization we can listen to and create new thoughts that could lead to a sense of wholeness and well-being.

One person with AIDS told us, "I can remember when I first heard the notion of alternative therapies. I thought and felt the whole thing was nonsense. I have since discovered that it's really important to keep an open mind. I went from feeling complete contempt for the mumbo-jumbo of alternative therapies to incorporating these same therapies in my daily life."

SUGGESTED READING

Cousins, Norman. 1985. *Anatomy of An Illness As Perceived by the Patient*. New York: Bantam Books.

Crook, William. 1986. *The Yeast Connection*. New York: Vintage Books.

Fox, Emmet. 1950. *Alter Your Life*. New York: Harper & Row.

Gawain, Shakti. 1982. *Creative Visualization*. New York: Bantam Books.

Gawain, Shakti. *Living in the Light*. 1986. San Rafael, CA: Whatever Publications.

Justice, Blair. 1987. *Who Gets Sick?* Los Angeles: St. Martin's Press.

Krishnamurti, J. 1972. *You Are the World*. New York: Harper & Row.

Levine, Stephen. 1984. *Meeting At the Edge*. Garden City, NY: Anchor Books.

Pearsall, Paul. 1987. *Superimmunity*. New York: McGraw-Hill.

Peck, M. Scott. 1978. *The Road Less Traveled*. New York: Simon & Schuster.

Weiner, Michael. 1986. *Maximum Immunity*. Boston: Houghton Mifflin.

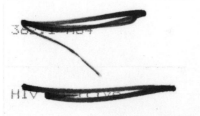